ILLUSTRATED ELEMENTS OF

NUTRITIONAL
HEALING

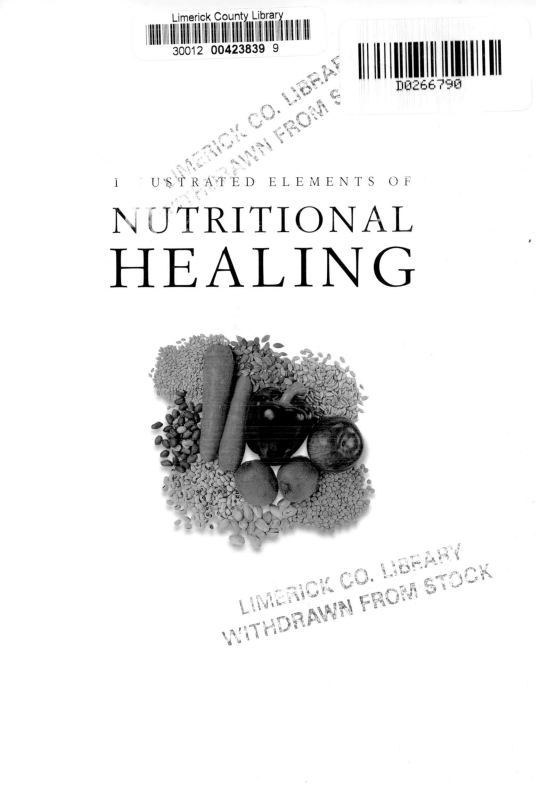

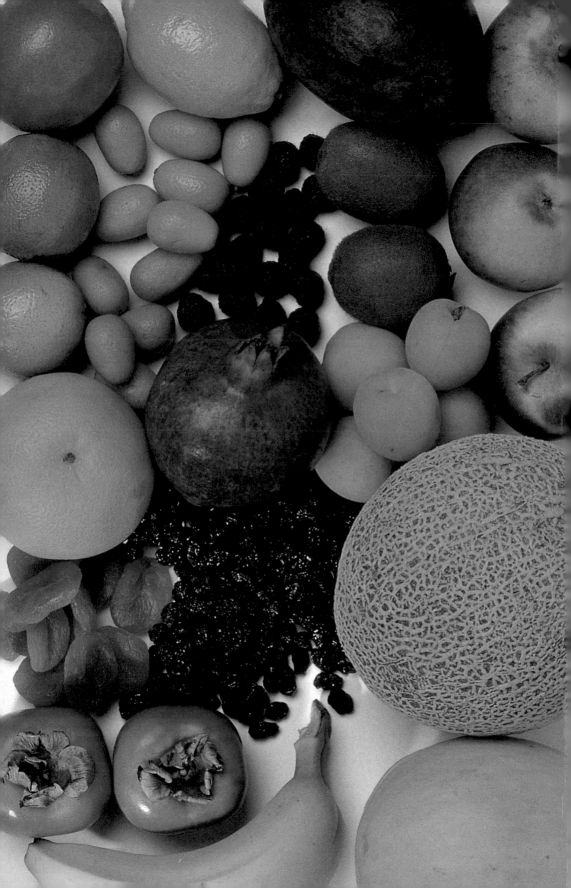

ILLUSTRATED ELEMENTS OF
NUTRITIONAL
HEALING

DENISE MORTIMORE

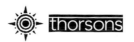

For Lucy and Tom, my source of inspiration.

Thorsons
An imprint of HarperCollins*Publishers*
77–85 Fulham Palace Road
Hammersmith, London W6 8JB

The Thorsons website address is www.thorsons.com

THORSONS is a trademark™ of HarperCollins*Publishers*

First published in Great Britain in 2003 by Thorsons

2 4 6 8 10 9 7 5 3 1

Text copyright © Denise Mortimore 2003
Copyright © HarperCollins*Publishers* Ltd 2003

Denise Mortimore asserts the moral right to
be identified as the author of this work

The book was created by THE BRIDGEWATER BOOK COMPANY

A catalogue record for this book
is available from the British Library

ISBN 0 00 713688 9

Printed and bound in Hong Kong by Printing Express.

NOTE FROM THE PUBLISHER
The information given in this book is not
intended to be taken as a replacement for medical
advice. Any person with a condition requiring
medical treatment should consult a qualified practitioner.

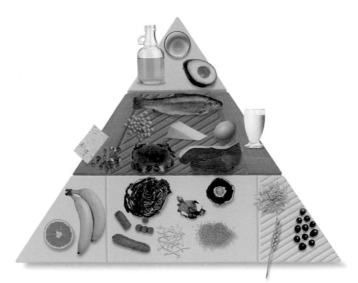

Contents

Introduction

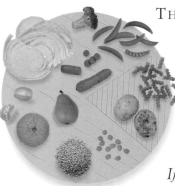

THE HUMAN BODY *is a complex biochemical machine that has specific requirements for health. In addition to proteins, fats, carbohydrates, energy, and water, there are some 40 different vitamins, minerals, essential fatty acids, amino acids, and other components needed by our body for it to remain healthy. We also need oxygen (from air), warmth, shelter, sunlight, and companionship. If we are deprived of any of these, we soon wither.*

ABOVE *The advantages of nutritional healing include an improvement in general health and a sense of well-being.*

A deficiency in any one of the essential nutrients will result in anything from mild, almost imperceptible, ill-health through a wide range of symptoms and diseases to eventual death. Multiple deficiencies are common in individuals who eat a typical Western diet, characterized by its many excesses alongside its lack of essential nutrients, leading to biochemical chaos.

Nutrient-deficient diets and those which also include large and frequent amounts of common allergens (wheat, yeast, milk, eggs, citrus, alcohol, etc.) can impair digestion, irritate the gut lining, and lead to a range of food intolerances in susceptible people. Suboptimum nutrition, especially if further compromised by an unhealthy lifestyle of insufficient exercise, smoking, high stress levels, and lack of proper rest and relaxation, may eventually take us along the road to chronic ill-health and degenerative disease.

Complementary medicines and health practices, such as nutritional therapy, are becoming the natural choice of growing numbers of people. Anyone who is willing to undertake changes in eating habits and lifestyle, and stick to them, will reap manifold the rewards of their work. There is absolutely nothing to lose and everything to gain.

ABOVE *Nutritional therapy is not just for adults; even young children can reap the benefits.*

How to Use this Book

You have picked up this book because you think that there is room for improvement in your life. You may be feeling a little tired and "run down"; you may have members of your family who are ill; perhaps you are troubled by niggling symptoms or you are chronically sick. *Illustrated Elements of Nutritional Healing* will give you a general idea of the basic principles that are at the foundation of nutritional therapy, explaining what is really meant by the term "balanced diet". Self-assessment questionnaires will help you to identify specific health problems. Finally, beneficial foods and supplements are listed for many conditions.

BELOW **The first few chapters of the book introduce you to the principles of nutritional healing, and examine the whole concept of optimum nutrition and a "balanced diet".**

BELOW **The Common Ailment section of the book enables you to carry out self-assessment questionnaires that will lead you to a greater understanding of how to regain and organize your health.**

Diagrams and tables help to explain the nutritional values of the different food groups.

Simple questionnaires will help you take an analytical view of certain disorders, and will lead you toward the correct nutritional program.

The main text explains the origins of common disorders and suggests ways of modifying your diet to help deal with the causes.

RIGHT **The final chapters of the book are devoted to specific conditions that are likely to be helped by nutritional healing.**

The main text examines the body's primary systems in detail and highlights potential health problems.

Each complaint is accompanied by a diet recommending foods that should form the bulk of your nutritional program, together with helpful food supplements.

What is Nutritional Healing?

ABOVE *The daily consumption of fresh fruit is an essential part of a healthy diet.*

NUTRITIONAL HEALING *works on a principle that is so simple that it is generally overlooked: that what you absorb into your body must affect how it functions. "You are what you eat" is obviously not the whole truth, but what you eat cannot help but contribute to how you are. Nutritional healing is a practical way of overcoming illness and promoting health naturally without the use of toxic drugs.*

During nutritional healing the whole body heals itself so that:

❖ the cause of the disease is treated and not just the symptoms;

❖ additional health problems are addressed simultaneously;

❖ general health is improved and opportunistic infections are prevented.

As with all reputable therapies, the holistic and individual approach is vital. Any person truly wishing to improve his or her state of health will want to encourage healing in the "whole" body and not just the part of it that is presently malfunctioning. Also, since each person has a body chemistry that is unique to them (arising from their unique genetic inheritance, their constitution, and their particular environment), it is obvious that each individual must be treated according to his or her own symptoms. This treatment is likely to be quite different from that given to another individual who would usually be diagnosed as having the same disease. Nevertheless, the initial stages involved in loss of health are caused in nearly all cases by several common factors.

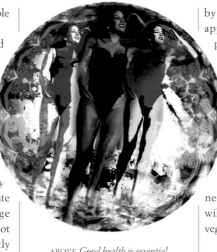

ABOVE *Good health is essential to our well-being and underpins our whole enjoyment of life.*

Nutritional healing bases its success in five main areas of dietary change (see opposite). Dietary improvements can be introduced gradually at your own pace and fitted into your lifestyle. A gradual change in diet leads to greater success and a more permanent improvement in health. Rapid changes in diet are unlikely to be sustained. The gradual approach means that the benefits of nutritional healing do not occur as rapidly as treatment given by a more conventional medical approach, and some degree of patience is required .

Nutritional Healing has nothing to do with "fad" diets, and there is no need to be a "health freak" to partake of this natural system of healing. Moreover it is a lifelong approach to eating that you will be happy to follow. Vegetarianism is an option but not a necessity, though all healing diets will contain optimum amounts of vegetables and fruit.

The timescale for improvement of health by change in diet depends on many things; for example, how long you have had the symptoms, how committed you are to your new regime, the types and quality of the supplements you use, and the improvement in other areas of your lifestyle. In general, you should begin to reap the benefits in two to four weeks. In some cases of deeply entrenched ill-health it may take a little longer, since repair of digestive function, removing toxins, and nourishing the body properly require time. But if you persevere, your sense of well-being will reach new heights.

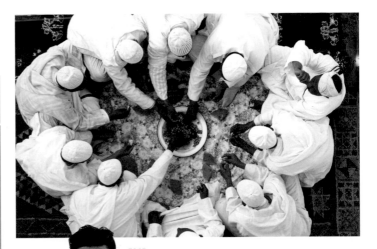

RIGHT *Men gather together to share locally produced foods in Morocco.*

FIVE RULES FOR RESTORING HEALTH

The nutritional therapist's five ground rules for restoring the body to health are:

1 Correct faulty digestion and eliminate food intolerances by combining appropriate foods, and by observing reactions to different food groups.

2 Decrease toxic overload by increasing the amount of nutritious, organic food, and decreasing the amount of rich and overprocessed foods.

3 Release healing energy for elimination of toxins by making balanced choices from foods that are part of your food culture.

4 Rebalance the intestinal bacteria in order to encourage conditions that improve absorption of important minerals, vitamins, amino acids, essential fatty acids, and other components.

5 Identify and support weakened, overburdened, or exhausted organs by correct supplementation.

BELOW *Healthy food is low in fats and high in nutrients.*

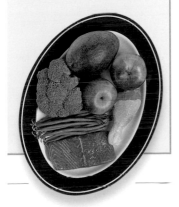

POOR NUTRITION LEADS TO MUSCLE FATIGUE

FOOD INTOLERANCE CAN MANIFEST ITSELF IN HEADACHES

FOOD CULTURE

On this planet there are billions of people consuming different diets and experiencing different disease patterns. It is likely that the longer a group of people maintain their "cultural" diet the more individuals will adapt to it, as long as the diet contains a balanced range of basic nutrients and little "chemical" interference. A high salt intake, for example, is not always associated with high blood pressure.

Our cultural roots, therefore, dictate to some degree the type of basic diet on which we thrive. The pattern of eating foods related to our own origins has been seriously eroded within the last three or four decades. This rapid change in basic diet, coupled with new methods of food production, preparation, and preservation, has been the main reason for decreasing standards of general health and fitness in the West. Individual biochemical differences are now playing a much greater part in the see-saw balance of our general health.

LEFT *Releasing toxins and rebalancing intestinal bacteria can quickly restore health and vitality.*

A Deficient Diet

IT IS FOOLISH to assume that giving any animal species a diet differing from the one it consumed during the major part of its evolution will not result in health problems. But this has happened in the West over the last century and we are paying the price.

MODERN DIET AND ITS IMBALANCES

In spite of the megabillions of dollars and pounds spent on health care, degenerative diseases are still on the increase in the West. By using proper nutrition and maintaining a healthier lifestyle, many of these diseases would be preventable, and, perhaps even curable.

For example, each year many millions of people die from cardiovascular diseases, including heart disease, arterial damage, and high blood pressure. The underlying causes of these diseases are more likely to be related to poor diet, insufficient exercise, a stressful lifestyle, and toxins – environmental pollutants, tobacco, drugs, and alcohol – than anything else.

Large-scale food processing, for example the refining of flour, can be detrimental to the nutritional quality of food. When flour is refined, the

---

WESTERN DIET

Simply put, the typical Western diet contains:

✿ Too much animal fat but insufficient good-quality essential fatty acids

✿ Too much "salt" but an insufficient range and amount of mineral salts

✿ Too much sugar and refined carbohydrate products but insufficient fiber

✿ Too many processed foods with consequent vitamin loss

✿ Too many stimulants: tea, coffee, and alcohol

✿ Too much alcohol

---

dietary fiber, essential vitamins, and minerals, which are needed by the body to turn starchy food into energy, are removed. Highly processed convenience foods, full of artificial flavorings and colors, have now flooded onto the market. Many food additives can be harmful to susceptible individuals. In addition, most food additives have not been tested in groups, and therefore their synergistic effects are unknown.

It has been said that people in the West are overfed and undernourished – although many people's total energy intake is excessive, the quality of food is often so poor that the nutrient intake in terms of vitamins and minerals is inadequate. This is in contrast to some developing countries where there simply is not sufficient food of any kind to sustain basic life.

Many of the diseases of the West have been linked with excessive fat, sugar, or salt. However, the additional problems of overprocessed and nutrient-deficient food, combined with a widespread incidence of deficient digestion and poor assimilation of nutrients, is yet to be recognized fully.

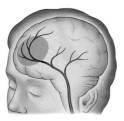

ABOVE *Damage to the frontal area of the brain is caused by circulatory disorders.*

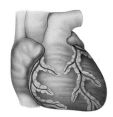

ABOVE *Excess cholesterol can block an artery in the heart, which destroys heart muscle.*

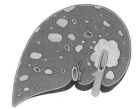

ABOVE *Cancerous tissue – the lighter areas – in a cross-section of the liver.*

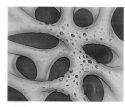

ABOVE *A lack of calcium in the diet leads to osteoporosis.*

KIDNEY BEANS – DRYING BEANS HAS LONG BEEN A NATURAL FORM OF PRESERVATION

SUNFLOWER SEEDS, A GOOD SOURCE OF ESSENTIAL FATTY ACIDS

EGGPLANT (AUBERGINE) IS A RELATIVE NEWCOMER TO MOST DIETS

WALNUTS – NUTS HAVE ALWAYS FEATURED IN THE HUMAN DIET

OATS ARE ONE OF THE MOST NUTRITIOUS GRAINS

ABOVE *A modern healthy diet can be built around the same types of nutritious foods to which we have adapted during the course of our evolution.*

SWEET PEPPERS ARE VERY HIGH IN VITAMIN C

BROWN RICE STILL HAS THE ROUGHAGE THAT HAS BEEN REMOVED FROM WHITE RICE

DIET AND EVOLUTION

Early Humans (25,000 B.C.E.) Around 50,000 years ago our diet consisted of meat, nuts, fruit, and berries. As the animals eaten were wild and free to roam, their meat was lean.

Hunter–Gatherers (10,000 B.C.E.) With the development of agriculture, humans began to cultivate and develop grains and keep animals for consumption of their milk.

The Middle Ages (1500) In Europe the range of vegetables increased and consumption of both freshwater and saltwater fish become more widespread.

Present Day The range of foods an individual can eat is limited only by preference and by the size of his or her budget. Refined sugar, hydrogenated fat, high-fat meats, dairy food, salt, pastry, white flour, diet drinks, coffee, and "convenience" foods have become dietary staples.

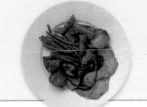

OUR FUTURE IS ON OUR PLATE

Blatantly bad nutrition quickly brings about serious clinical symptoms. However, in Western society our marginal diet more commonly encourages subclinical deficiencies that do not surface as diagnosable problems until years have passed. A person with no symptoms but with abnormally high cholesterol in their blood, for example, is at risk of eventually developing heart disease. A person with no symptoms but abnormally high platelet aggregation (stickiness of blood cells) is at greater risk of suffering a stroke or a circulatory disorder. A person with low tissue and blood calcium and other minerals is at greater risk of developing osteoporosis.

What people eat today may not affect them now, but it is likely to affect them greatly in the future.

Cumulative poor nutrition creates diseases that are not recognized as nutrition-related disorders. But this is exactly what they are. Long-term subclinical deficiency of vitamin C may produce anything from heart disease to gallstones. Long-term subclinical deficiency of chromium and zinc may bring about poor glucose tolerance and blood-sugar problems later in life.

Nutritional therapists believe that an adequate intake of vitamin E and essential fatty acids, among other nutrients, can help to prevent heart disease, lung damage from air pollution, cancer, and premenstrual syndrome. Modern research is now confirming that long-term vitamin deficiencies may surface as common degenerative diseases, such as heart disease and cancer, rather than simply being associated with specific problems, such as scurvy.

Optimum Nutrition and Super Nutrition

ABOVE *Extra vitamin E can be very beneficial.*

MODERN LIVING *brings with it pollutants in air and water, additives in food, and toxic chemicals. These substances are, in the greater part, "foreign" materials. They are likely to put an increased demand on our metabolism because they have to be rendered harmless and eliminated. Potentially, therefore, we require even greater amounts of the essential nutrients than we ever did before.*

In addition to combating pollution and stress with an optimum intake of nutrients, some people's nutrient requirements are above average. Inherited defects in metabolism, advancing age, excessive exercise, illnesses, pregnancy, and lactation; all of these factors, plus others, may also elevate nutrient needs.

Nutritional therapists believe that certain nutrients taken at high levels can become "disease-beaters" and develop "supernutrient" powers.

For example, 12–18mg niacin (vitamin B₃) per day is the reference nutrient intake (R.N.I.) for general health, but when five or more times that amount is consumed, niacin becomes an effective dilator of blood vessels. These large doses of niacin can normalize the levels of fats in the blood, which may help people who have had heart attacks or who are at risk, genetically, from furring up of the arteries. Extremely high doses of vitamin A and vitamin

C (only under supervision) help to protect the body against the destructive (but potentially helpful) effect of chemotherapy. High doses of vitamin E (400–800IU per day) reduce breast tenderness in premenstrual women, as well as thinning

BELOW *Modern life, with its relentless pace, its constant emphasis on consumption, its pollution, and its ready use of chemical cures for all ailments, leaves us subject to many stress-induced illnesses.*

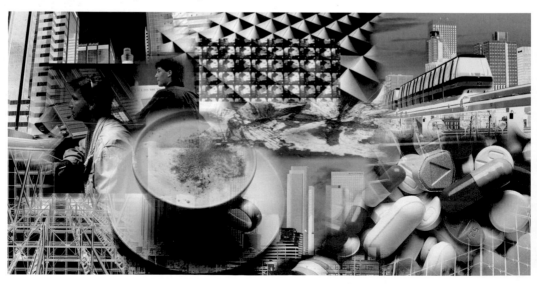

the blood and improving circulation in individuals with circulatory disorders. High doses of zinc (15–30mg per day) and vitamin C (1–3g per day) boost immune function and wound healing.

Thus "normal" levels of nutrients may be different for different people depending on many factors of their lifestyle and state of health, sex, and age. In fact, "normal amounts" of nutrients will be those levels which are sufficient to maintain "normal" health, while nutritional therapists believe above-normal amounts of nutrients appear to have "super-nutrient" abilities and can be used in extreme heal ing situations.

Nutritional support can also increase the effectiveness of more conventional health treatment such as drugs, surgery, and cancer therapy. Many aggressive procedures create stress in the body and elevate nutrient needs at a time when the patient is less likely to eat well.

Optimum nutrition can also prevent future disease by elevating a person from subclinical deficiency into a healthy "saturation" state for all essential nutrients. Therefore, optimum nutrition, and in some instances super nutrition, will raise many people from an average health status to a more elevated level of physical and mental well-being.

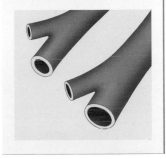

EFFECTS OF NIACIN

Vitamin B₃ (niacin) taken at five times the level usually needed helps dilate clogged-up blood vessels, which is useful to those with coronary disease.

BELOW LEFT *Normal blood vessel*
BELOW RIGHT *Dilated blood vessel*

CLEAR EYES SHOW PLENTY OF ENERGY

SHINY HAIR

A GOOD COMPLEXION

STRONG TEETH

FRESH-LOOKING SKIN

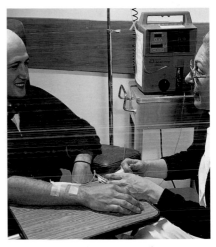

ABOVE *Extra vitamins and minerals are often advisable for patients, such as this man undergoing chemotherapy.*

LEFT *Good health is apparent in the body's whole appearance.*

Personal Nutritional Status

TO ESTABLISH YOUR *optimum nutrient intake, you must consider the factors that determine how much nutrition your body is getting, such as the quality of your diet and the efficiency of your digestion. Your unique needs are also influenced by factors such as age, gender, and stress.*

THE QUALITY OF FOOD

Food grown on poor soil can be deficient in certain nutrients and contaminated with pesticides or chemical fertilizers. Livestock may only have access to contaminated foods and may be treated with drugs such as antibiotics, and growth enhancers. The only way to insure your food is not contaminated in this way is to consume organic produce. If this is problematic, reduce the chemical load on your body by washing all vegetables and fruit thoroughly, and having less meat and dairy produce in your diet.

THE TYPE OF FOOD

Nutrient-dense foods such as vegetables, fruit, pulses (legumes), wholegrains, fish, nuts, and seeds improve the nutritional status of the person who eats them. The results of several scientific studies now confirm that eating a diet high in nutrients but low in calorific content helps prevent signs of aging, and increases lifespan.

DIGESTION

An individual whose digestive system is inefficient is more likely to have a poor nutritional status than someone with efficient digestion. Inefficient digestive systems may be

FACTORS AFFECTING NUTRITIONAL STATUS

There are four main factors that influence nutritional status:
❀ the quality of the food we eat
❀ the quantity of the food we eat
❀ the efficiency of the whole digestive process
❀ biochemical individuality (see page 15).

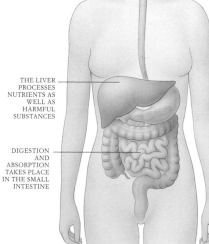

RIGHT *Food undergoes a complex process of digestion, absorption, and assimilation.*

FOOD IS PROPELLED THROUGH THE ESOPHAGUS

THE LIVER PROCESSES NUTRIENTS AS WELL AS HARMFUL SUBSTANCES

DIGESTION AND ABSORPTION TAKES PLACE IN THE SMALL INTESTINE

caused by insufficient production of hydrochloric acid in the stomach, or poor digestive enzyme production by the pancreas and other enzyme-secreting glands.

ABSORPTION

If for some reason the end products of digestion are not being absorbed properly, because of poor membrane function, intestinal irritation, or a condition such as celiac disease, then the nutritional status of that individual will be compromised. Some substances in the diet, for example tea, coffee, and certain types of fiber, can reduce the absorption of nutrients such as iron and zinc.

ASSIMILATION

The efficiency with which nutrients are used by the body can also have an effect upon nutritional status. Some individuals have metabolic faults (as a result of a genetic defect, food intolerance, other nutritional deficiencies, food toxins, and environmental pollutants) that prevent the body from efficiently utilizing nutrients.

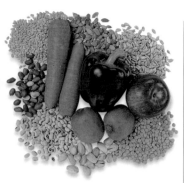

ABOVE *Fruit, vegetables, nuts, and grains are rich in nutrients, especially if produced organically.*

BIOCHEMICAL INDIVIDUALITY

Individual biochemical makeup is a fundamental concept in understanding the factors that determine whether a person remains healthy or becomes sick. Our individual nutritional requirements are influenced by a number of factors.

AGE

As we age, we may need greater amounts of essential nutrients both to combat the wear and tear of an aging metabolism and digestive system, and to counteract the nutrient-depleting effect of medication. Conversely calorific intake needs to be reduced as we age.

GENDER

Nutrient requirements are different between men and women, and even between boys and girls. In addition, they may vary throughout a woman's menstrual cycle.

GROWTH

Young children have different nutritional requirements from adults. Protein, essential fatty acids, and

---

SEVEN STEPS TO HEALTHY EATING

1 Eat a "culturally based" diet of fish, shellfish, game, lean meats, seeds, nuts, fruit, roots, leaves, and whole grains.

2 Eat nutrient-dense food to combat present ill-health and to protect against future disease.

3 Guard against overeating of carbohydrates and fats.

4 Eat organic food and drink filtered, distilled, or bottled water whenever possible to cut down on intake of pollutants.

5 Remove as many environmental pollutants as possible.

6 Avoid processed food, refined food, and food additives, and replace them with wholefoods.

7 Cut down on stimulants (tea, coffee, salt, sugar, and soft drinks) as well as alcohol.

---

certain minerals, such as zinc, are required in greater amounts by children at puberty than by adults.

PREGNANCY AND LACTATION

A woman who is pregnant or breastfeeding needs to take in increased amounts of minerals such as calcium, magnesium, and zinc, as well as insure an optimum intake of beta-carotene and vitamins A, B, C, E.

STATE OF GENERAL HEALTH

Many conditions severely deplete resources of certain nutrients: for example, protein loss (loss of amino acids) after surgery; zinc and vitamin C loss after extensive skin burns. However, force-feeding a sick person can put his or her metabolism under greater stress. Eating to "keep your strength up" is not always the best advice.

STRESS

Certain types of stress may increase requirements of some nutrients, such as the B-complex of vitamins.

ACTIVITY LEVEL

Anyone who exercises frequently may have an increased requirement for iron and zinc. Since the metabolism is enhanced by exercise, general nutrient requirement will be increased.

DRUGS AND TOXIC LEVELS

Any person on prescribed or recreational drugs, or living and working in a polluted environment, will find their nutritional requirements greatly increased because the body needs help to detoxify these chemicals. Even tea- and coffee-drinking can increase nutrient requirements.

LEFT *A pregnant woman should take increased amounts of minerals.*

How Nutritional Imbalances Lead to Disease

MUCH OF THE *information available in the media would have us believe that vitamins are the all-important dietary factor for good health, whereas, although vitamins are important for an efficient metabolism, minerals and trace elements are at least as important and in some cases more important in the workings of our biochemistry. Nutritional therapists believe that suboptimum nutrition can impair the body's ability to retain essential minerals.*

Despite the chemical similarity of certain pairs of minerals, such as calcium and magnesium, and sodium and potassium, their biochemical activity is very different. This is illustrated by the fact that most body cells actively collect potassium and excrete sodium, and similarly, many actively import magnesium and export calcium. The first step along the road to poor health seems to originate in body tissues failing in this basic "separation" principle, which leads to acidity (or toxemia) of the tissues. There are parts of the body where the environment needs to be acid: the stomach, for the digestion of food; the colon for microbial balance and nutrient absorption; the skin for bacterial control. But in all other areas the acidity/alkalinity of the tissues should remain neutral, or within a very narrow range around it.

As nutrient intake falls below optimum, nutritional therapists believe that the general ability of body cells to retain a range of nutrients, and especially minerals, within the cell, and to remove others to different areas, starts to fail. Energy levels drop and tissues become more acid (toxic), which in turn reduces the acidity of those areas which need to be acid. If, for example, the acidity of the stomach is reduced, then

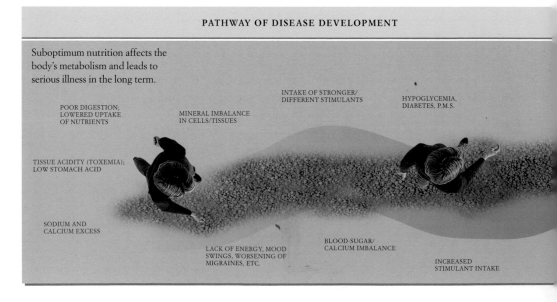

PATHWAY OF DISEASE DEVELOPMENT

Suboptimum nutrition affects the body's metabolism and leads to serious illness in the long term.

POOR DIGESTION;
LOWERED UPTAKE
OF NUTRIENTS

MINERAL IMBALANCE
IN CELLS/TISSUES

INTAKE OF STRONGER/
DIFFERENT STIMULANTS

HYPOGLYCEMIA,
DIABETES, P.M.S.

TISSUE ACIDITY (TOXEMIA);
LOW STOMACH ACID

SODIUM AND
CALCIUM EXCESS

LACK OF ENERGY, MOOD
SWINGS, WORSENING OF
MIGRAINES, ETC.

BLOOD-SUGAR/
CALCIUM IMBALANCE

INCREASED
STIMULANT INTAKE

food, and particularly protein, will not be broken down to a suitable state for digestive enzymes to act upon it in the small intestine. As undigested or partly digested food travels through the gut, it will irritate certain areas, prevent the uptake of digested end products and encourage the wrong type of bacteria and other micro-organisms in the bowel. The overall effect is then a decrease in body energy, an inefficient metabolism, and the beginnings of malfunction.

If, at the same time, the diet contains too much sodium (from "salt" and convenience foods) and calcium, it is likely that cellular imbalance and the degree of tissue acidity may be further encouraged. The first signs that something is wrong are lack of energy, mood swings, and the worsening of any existing condition like migraine or asthma. Underlying these symptoms is a change in the body's regulatory mechanisms so that blood-sugar control and calcium metabolism become unbalanced. As symptoms worsen, we find ourselves attracted to stronger and different stimulants, such as sugar, salt, refined foods, alcohol, tea, and coffee. The body becomes even less capable of good maintenance, and a subtle collection of minor symptoms becomes disease. As the downward spiral continues, hormonal glands can become over-stressed, leading to adrenal and pancreatic exhaustion and, ultimately, to the failure of the immune and endocrine systems.

ACIDITY

Acidity/alkalinity levels should be balanced throughout most of the body.

A healthy body is one where acidity and alkalinity are appropriate to that part of the body.

Poor health comes from too little acid in the stomach or colon or too much in other bodily tissue.

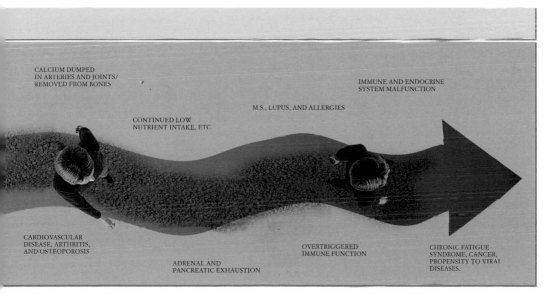

CALCIUM DUMPED IN ARTERIES AND JOINTS/ REMOVED FROM BONES

IMMUNE AND ENDOCRINE SYSTEM MALFUNCTION

M.S., LUPUS, AND ALLERGIES

CONTINUED LOW NUTRIENT INTAKE, ETC.

CARDIOVASCULAR DISEASE, ARTHRITIS, AND OSTEOPOROSIS

OVERTRIGGERED IMMUNE FUNCTION

CHRONIC FATIGUE SYNDROME, CANCER, PROPENSITY TO VIRAL DISEASES.

ADRENAL AND PANCREATIC EXHAUSTION

What is a Well-balanced Diet?

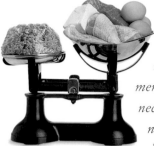

THE OLD BELIEF *that as long as you eat foods from the four main food groups (meats, dairy foods, fruit/vegetables, and carbohydrates) and eat three good "square" meals a day, you are receiving all the nutrients you need, is inadequate. It makes no mention of the types and variety of foods within each group that are necessary for a healthy balance; it does not recognize the possible nutrient depletion in "processed foods", and takes no account of the biochemical uniqueness, changing needs, or state of health of the individual. When you have a clear understanding of your own dietary needs, you should be able to formulate your own eating plan.*

ABOVE *Conventional advice about balanced diets takes no account of the acid/alkali balance in the body, which is vital for good health.*

Because of modern food-production and preservation techniques, even fruit and vegetables do not contain the levels of nutrients they did in the past. Analysis of nutrient levels has indicated, on average, a decline of around 22 percent in mineral content of fruit and vegetables over the last 50 years. It has even been found that some supermarket oranges contain no vitamin C whatsoever.

Surveys carried out in Britain on tens of thousands of people have indicated that more than seven in every ten people are borderline deficient or severely deficient in B vitamins. Nutrition reviews carried out in 1992 demonstrated that it is impossible to get sufficient vitamins from the regular American food supply.

Furthermore, nutritional therapists believe that many modern diseases have their basis in acidosis (toxemia) of the tissues. Very small changes in pH (acid/alkali balance) of the blood to the order of 0.01 pH points appear to make a significant difference to a person's health. The healthy norm is pH 7.46, with 7.49 being extremely alkaline and pH 7.40 being extremely acid. However, conventional medical authorities

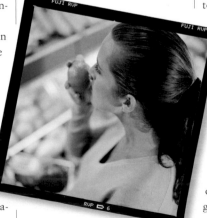

ABOVE *Fruit and vegetables have declined in nutritional value.*

continue to maintain that nutrition does not play a part in the acid/alkali balance of the body because they consider the normal range of blood pH to be 7.4 to 7.5. Even wide fluctuations in eating patterns are unlikely to produce scores outside this range.

Under normal conditions, symptoms of over-acidity (poor mental function, fatigue, arthritic disorders, muscle aches and pains, and so on) should not occur because the body is able to "buffer" any excess acid via alkaline reserves in blood and bone. Modern living, however, can exhaust this capacity. For example, meat is a very concentrated source of protein and if eaten two times a day over a period of several days it can generate a state of acidity that has to be neutralized by, primarily, the bicarbonate buffer system. This requires sodium and calcium.

When blood reserves are used up, the body calls on calcium from the bones. This link between excessive protein consumption and bone-density loss puts a very large question mark over the necessity for large amounts of protein in a healthy diet. However, a healthy diet must contain sufficient protein to meet bodily demands, and this needs to be balanced adequately with complex carbohydrates.

Another example is where alcohol, which is detoxified by the liver, is taken in excess. It overwhelms the detoxifying enzyme systems in the liver, and instead of alcohol being metabolized to carbon dioxide and water it is converted to acetaldehyde. This is an extremely toxic substance and gives rise to "ketoacidosis", which manifests itself as a hangover, putting an even greater strain on the acid/alkali balancing system. Since these acid-buffering systems depend on a sufficient supply of alkaline minerals, it is imperative that our diets contain enough foods to supply these.

We also need to know the difference between the natural acidity of a food and its ability to become "acid-forming". When a food is metabolized, a mineral "ash" remains and when this ash is rich in calcium, magnesium, sodium, and potassium, it is "alkali-forming", but when the ash contains large amounts of chlorine, phosphorus, and sulfur it becomes "acid-forming". To counteract the tendency toward acidosis and its ensuing symptoms, the diet needs to be made up of 80 percent alkali-forming foods, and only 20 percent acid-forming foods. This recommendation is not even hinted at in conventional advice about "balanced diets".

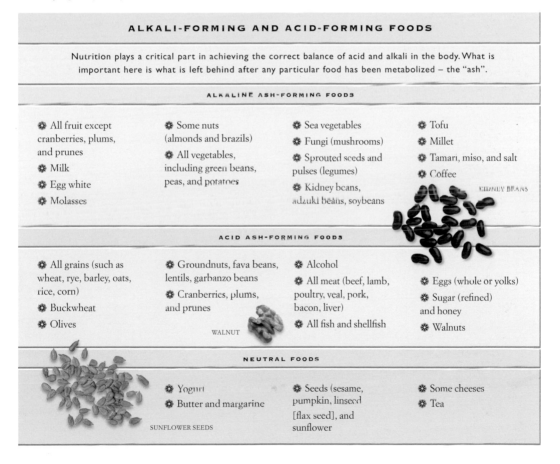

ALKALI-FORMING AND ACID-FORMING FOODS

Nutrition plays a critical part in achieving the correct balance of acid and alkali in the body. What is important here is what is left behind after any particular food has been metabolized – the "ash".

ALKALINE ASH-FORMING FOODS

* All fruit except cranberries, plums, and prunes
* Milk
* Egg white
* Molasses
* Some nuts (almonds and brazils)
* All vegetables, including green beans, peas, and potatoes
* Sea vegetables
* Fungi (mushrooms)
* Sprouted seeds and pulses (legumes)
* Kidney beans, adzuki beans, soybeans
* Tofu
* Millet
* Tamari, miso, and salt
* Coffee

KIDNEY BEANS

ACID ASH-FORMING FOODS

* All grains (such as wheat, rye, barley, oats, rice, corn)
* Buckwheat
* Olives
* Groundnuts, fava beans, lentils, garbanzo beans
* Cranberries, plums, and prunes
* Alcohol
* All meat (beef, lamb, poultry, veal, pork, bacon, liver)
* All fish and shellfish
* Eggs (whole or yolks)
* Sugar (refined) and honey
* Walnuts

WALNUT

NEUTRAL FOODS

* Yogurt
* Butter and margarine
* Seeds (sesame, pumpkin, linseed [flax seed], and sunflower
* Some cheeses
* Tea

SUNFLOWER SEEDS

The New Food Pyramid Program

EVERY MEAL SHOULD *be a balance of carbohydrate, protein, and essential fatty acids, and at the same time attempt to achieve 80 percent alkali-forming and neutral foods to 20 percent acid-forming foods. The tables on page 22 should give you a rough guide to help you achieve a healthy balance of foods.*

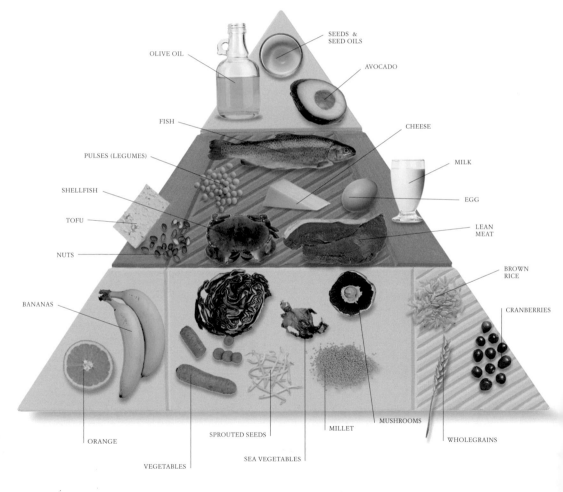

SEEDS & SEED OILS

OLIVE OIL

AVOCADO

FISH

CHEESE

PULSES (LEGUMES)

MILK

SHELLFISH

EGG

TOFU

LEAN MEAT

NUTS

BROWN RICE

BANANAS

CRANBERRIES

ORANGE

SPROUTED SEEDS

MILLET

MUSHROOMS

WHOLEGRAINS

VEGETABLES

SEA VEGETABLES

ABOVE *The space given to a food in the pyramid indicates how much of the diet should come from each of the food groups to promote good health.*

CARBOHYDRATES

At the base of the pyramid, and therefore making up the largest portion of your food, are the fruit, vegetables, and wholegrain carbohydrates. They should constitute around 40 percent of your calorie intake. Bear in mind that refined carbohydrates (white bread, sugar, sugar-rich cakes and cookies, pastries) have no place here. Grains (including bread, pasta, rice, millet, breakfast cereals, buckwheat etc.) and starchy vegetables need to be kept at a low to moderate level to prevent blood- sugar imbalances.

PROTEINS

The middle level contains the proteins. These should make up around 30 percent of your calorie intake.

TREATS

A diet without any treats is not going to be adhered to for very long and the odd cake, chocolate, or glass of wine is going to do you no harm, but bear in mind that the health-giving foods within this program are meant to become your major everyday choices.

Select a good range from (in descending order of importance) oily fish, lean meat, tofu, lentils, beans, seeds, nuts, milk, cheese, and eggs. Always have an equal balance of animal and plant protein if you are a meat eater, and for two or three days a week take your

protein quota from the pulses (legumes), seeds, nuts, and tofu. Insure that alkali-forming or neutral vegetable protein like tofu, almonds, brazil nuts, seeds, and pulses is balanced with the acid-forming proteins.

FATS AND OILS

The top of the pyramid accounts for around 30 percent of your calorie intake, but since fats and oils are high in calories, you need to make sure that you have very small servings. For example, if you are having a meal containing 3oz (75g) of fish (or tofu) plus a large salad, then your fat quota would be obtained from half a teaspoon of olive oil, or a few seeds. Seeds supply Omega-6 fatty acids; and pumpkin and linseed Omega-3 acids.

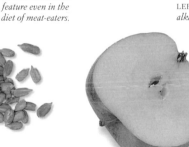

ABOVE *Oily fish is an excellent source of protein.*

RIGHT *Nuts should feature even in the diet of meat-eaters.*

LEFT *Most fruit is alkali-forming.*

COLOR KEY

- MONO-UNSATURATED AND POLYUNSATURATED FATS
- PROTEIN
- CARBOHYDRATES
- ACID-FORMING FOODS
- ACID-FORMING FOODS
- PLAIN BACKGROUNDS = ALKALI-FORMING/ "NEUTRAL" FOODS

ABOVE *Seeds are a source of fat to which our bodies are well adapted.*

BELOW *Green beans are a source of carbohydrate and fiber.*

BELOW *Though a fruit, avocado is a good source of essential fat.*

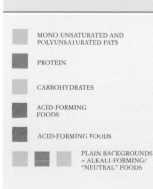

THE RESULTS OF THE NEW PYRAMID PROGRAM

Eating a diet constructed in the New Pyramid way will give your body ten major healthy changes.

❖ Saturated fat intake will be reduced, essential fatty acids raised.

❖ Protein levels, obtained from a range of sources, will be in line with the biochemical needs of the body.

❖ Sugar and salt intake will be reduced, and natural sugars and mineral salts will be obtained from vegetables and fruit.

❖ Intake of convenience foods and, therefore, intake of artificial additives, preservatives, excess sugars, and salt, will be decreased.

❖ Intake of all necessary vitamins and minerals will be greatly increased.

❖ Intake of important antioxidants and phytochemicals (biologically active chemicals in food that are not strictly classsified as nutrients) will be increased.

❖ Dietary fiber will be obtained from a range of fiber types.

❖ Carbohydrate intake will be well balanced and will consist of "complex" rather than "refined" types;

THE NEW PYRAMID SERVING SIZES

To establish your personal daily food requirements according to the New Pyramid program, refer to this table, which introduces you to how much food is meant by "one serving". Within the three basic food groups, there are various types of foods, and a specific weight of food is given for each type.

FOOD GROUP	FOOD		SERVING SIZE ONE
Carbohydrates	Vegetables – except potatoes;	C1	
	sprouted seeds; mushrooms	C1	4 ounces (100g)
	Fruit	C1	2 ounces (50g)
	Wholegrains and starchy		
	vegetables, e.g., potatoes	C2	1 ounce (27g)
Protein	Oily fish – includes 1 fat serving	P1	1½ ounces (40g)
	Shellfish	P1	1½ ounces (40g)
	Lean meat	P1	1 ounce (27g)
	Tofu	P1	3 ounces (80g)
	Dairy: cottage cheese	P1	2 ounces (50g)
	Hard cheese – includes 1 fat serving	P1	1 ounce (27g)
	Yogurt	P1	3 ounces (80g)
	Milk – non-fat	P1	3 ounces (80g)
	Eggs – includes 2 fat servings	P1	2 ounces (50g)
	Nuts – includes 2 fat servings	P2	1½ ounces (40g)
	Seeds – includes 1 fat serving	P2	2 ounces (50g)
	Pulses (legumes) – includes		
	1 carbohydrate serving	P2	2 ounces (50g)
Fats	Olive oil; sesame oil;		
	sunflower oil; butter	F1	½tsp (2.5ml)
	Nuts – includes some protein	F2	1tsp (5ml)
	Seeds – includes some protein	F2	1½tsp (7.5ml)
	Peanut butter; tahini		
	– includes some protein	F3	1tsp (5ml)
	Avocado	F3	1 ounce (27g)
	Fish oils – included in protein list		

grains will be at a low level and, correspondingly, any blood-sugar imbalances will be minimal.

❖ Intake of environmental toxins and pollutants will be drastically reduced if you consume most of your food from an organic source.

❖ The pH balance will conform more to the 80 percent alkaline/20 percent acid ratio.

When you embark on your New Food Pyramid program, you should remember that wholefoods taste different from processed foods, which contain all sorts of flavorings and flavor-enhancing chemicals. Moreover, the taste of food depends upon your ability to detect subtleties of flavor, which in turn depends upon the quality of your diet. This essentially means that as you change to the types of food recommended here, you may find them bland at first. However, after a week or two your palate will have cleared sufficiently for your taste buds to return to their natural state, and you will begin to enjoy the natural flavors of these chemical-free wholefoods. If you then eat any "flavor-enhanced" foods, you will experience an overpowering taste of salt and artificial flavors. Don't eat in a hurry, or when you are feeling stressed, and you will begin to really savor your food. Always chew your food thoroughly and drink plenty of water.

On the following pages a closer look at each of the food groups depicted in the New Food Pyramid shows the range of foods within each group and assesses the usefulness of the different types for improving and maintaining health.

RATIO OF DAILY SERVINGS

This table shows how the servings should be made up within each food group

NUMBER OF DAILY SERVINGS	CARBOHYDRATES		PROTEIN		OILS		
	c1	c2	p1	p2	F1	F2	F3
5	4	1	2	3	2	2	1
7	5	2	3	4	2	3	2
9	5	4*	5**	4	3	3	3
11	6	5*	6**	5	4	4	3

* As serving size increases, use more millet and potato to keep acidity low
** As serving size increases, use more tofu and/or fish to keep dairy foods low

DAILY SERVINGS

Related to body size and levels of activity

Small to average size	sedentary	5 servings of each group
Small to average size	moderately active	7 servings of each group
Small to average size	very active	9 servings of each group
Greater than average size	sedentary	7 servings of each group
Greater than average size	moderately active	9 servings of each group
Greater than average size	very active	11 servings of each group

GENERAL HINTS FOR THE NEW PYRAMID PROGRAM

❀ Avoid any form of sugar (except fructose); sugar-substitutes, refined, or processed food; food additives.

❀ Minimize alcohol, coffee, and tea. Drink herb, fruit or rooibosh tea; lactose-free dandelion coffee, or other grain coffee.

❀ Avoid fried (except stir-fried vegetables in a cold-pressed virgin olive oil), burned, or "browned" food, hydrogenated fats, and margarines. Use animal fat sparingly.

❀ Treat all fats, oils, and foods that contain them (nuts, seeds, etc.) with care, and ensure they are fresh.

❀ Eat organic, raw vegetables.

❀ Keep dairy foods to a minimum; they may be catarrh-forming. Swap cow's milk for rice milk, soy milk, or oat milk, and use soy cream instead of dairy cream. Eat live yogurt, any type, to replenish the natural gut flora.

❀ Drink four to six half-pint glasses of water per day, plus diluted fruit juices (1:1 juice to water), between meals **only** to prevent dilution of digestive enzymes. Keep citrus juices to a minimum.

❀ Supplement with a multivitamin/multimineral, and 1,000mg vitamin C.

Understanding Food Groups

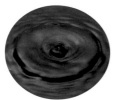

FOOD FALLS INTO *four major groups: fats, proteins, carbohydrates, and fiber. The other essential component of our diet is water. To eat properly you need to understand not only how these groups work together, but also the different categories within each group and their distinctive characteristics. A full understanding of the benefits, and problems, that characterize these food groups will enable you to make informed choices.*

ABOVE *Two-thirds of the body is made up of water, which is vital for life.*

FATS

There are basically two kinds of fats. Hard fats, which are solid at room temperature, usually come from an animal source such as fatty meat and dairy food (but also coconut), and are referred to as "saturated fats". Saturated fats are so called because all their chemical bonds are "saturated" with hydrogen atoms, and this tends to make molecules of this type of fat very rigid. Conversely, oils are "liquid" at room temperature. More often than not they come from a plant source, such as seeds and nuts (but also fish), and are referred to as "unsaturated" or "polyunsaturated" fats (oils). They are "unsaturated" because not all of the chemical bonds are linked to hydrogen atoms, which allows the formation of "double" bonds within the fat molecule, giving these oils a much more flexible structure.

BAD FATS

Animal fats (excluding fish oils), and in particular dairy foods, are high in saturated fat. Many of the degenerative diseases of modern humans (heart disease, stroke, obesity, M.S., and cancer) have been linked to our

SATURATED FATS

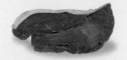

Dairy foods are high in saturated fat, though cottage cheese has much less than hard cheeses.

The increase in consumption of saturated fats is a contributory factor in the growth in heart disease.

Red meats can be made healthier by trimming off fat and broiling them so the fat drains away.

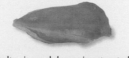

Poultry is much lower in saturated fats than beef, pork, or lamb.

large intake of saturated fat, which, because of its chemical nature, clogs up arteries and interferes with the body's metabolism. Additionally, saturated fat impedes the metabolism of good fats. It may also produce "insulin resistance", causing the blood-sugar control mechanism to fail.

You are rarely better off consuming "polyunsaturated" margarines or "low-fat" spreads because of the degree of processing these foods go through, in particular the process of "hydrogenation", where polyunsaturated oils are changed into solid or semi-solid fats.

Arachidonic acid, which interferes with hormonal control and immune function, and causes inappropriate clotting of the blood, is a fatty acid that can cause problems if taken in excess. Examples include offal, egg yolks, and fatty red meat.

Even unsaturated oils are chemically unstable and susceptible to damage by heat, light, oxygen, and metals. This instability can cause the production of "trans-fatty acids", which weaken the cell membranes, preventing the normal exchange of materials in and out of the cells.

GOOD FATS

Unsaturated fats (the so-called "good" fats) can be divided into two groups: mono-unsaturated fats, such as those found in olive oil; and polyunsaturated fats, such as those found in fish, nuts, and seeds. Mono-unsaturates appear to have a protective function against heart disease, as seen by the very good health of people living in the Mediterranean, while certain polyunsaturates are "essential". This means that the body cannot make them from other dietary fats or oils, so they must be taken into the body in their active form.

The two essential polyunsaturates are linoleic acid and linolenic acid. These belong to the Omega-6 and Omega-3 groups of oils respectively. Both are vital for the structure and effective working of the brain and nervous system, the immune system, the hormonal system, the cardiovascular system, and the skin.

The first indications of a deficiency in these two essential oils are dry skin, dry eyes, and a greater than normal thirst. Seeds in general, but especially sesame and sunflower seeds are rich in linoleic acid (Omega-6), while pumpkin and flax seeds (edible linseeds) are rich in linolenic acid (Omega-3).

Linoleic acid (Omega-6) is converted in the body into two further substances. These substances are known as gamma-linolenic acid (G.L.A.) and di-homo-gamma-linolenic acid (D.G.L.A.), which is further converted to arachidonic acid (A.A.). Linolenic acid (Omega-3) is converted to eicosapentaenoic acid (E.P.A.) and docosahexaenoic

acid (D.H.A.). E.P.A. and D.H.A. are also found in fatty fish (such as mackerel, herring, salmon, sardines, and so on).

Essential fatty acids (E.F.A.s) play a vital role in health, and you should therefore aim to have your full daily quota of essential fatty acids, found in cold-pressed olive oil, sesame seeds, sunflower seeds, pumpkin and linseeds, fish oils, evening primrose and borage flowers.

FATTY ACID PROFILE FOR VEGETABLE OILS

FRESH PRESSED ORGANIC OIL	SATURATED FAT	MONO-UNSATURATED	LINOLEIC	LINOLENIC
Almond	9%	65%	26%	-
Flax (linseed)	9%	16%	18%	57%
Hazelnut	7%	76%	17%	-
Olive	10%	82%	8%	-
Pumpkin	9%	34%	42%	15%
Safflower	8%	13%	79%	-
Sesame	13%	46%	41%	-
Sunflower	12%	19%	69%	-
Walnut	16%	28%	51%	5%

The above table is an extract from information obtained from Lamberts Healthcare Limited, England, with their kind permission.

BELOW *A vegetarian diet, especially one free of dairy produce and processed food, is very low in saturated fats.*

A DIET HIGH IN SEEDS AND NUTS RESULTS IN SHINY HAIR AND IMPROVED BRAIN FUNCTION

BROWN RICE AND VEGETABLES ARE HIGH IN NUTRIENTS AND LOW IN FAT

Understanding Cholesterol

FOR DECADES *we have been told that our blood cholesterol levels are related to our risk of heart disease, and the only way to reduce the risk is to cut cholesterol-containing foods from our diet. Fortunately, there is now much evidence to dispel these myths.*

Low-cholesterol diets actually encourage the liver to produce cholesterol while at the same time restricting many important nutrients (for example, the lecithin found in eggs), which are needed to control cholesterol levels in the body. Lecithin is a substance needed to emulsify fats and render fat molecules small enough to be carried efficiently in the blood to the cells, thereby removing them from the blood. People with atherosclerosis tend to produce small amounts of lecithin when compared to healthy people.

This may be because bodily production of lecithin needs essential fatty acids, choline, inositol, and magnesium, most of which tend to be low in low-cholesterol diets. Therefore, high blood cholesterol may be more related to lack of important nutrients, than directly to levels of cholesterol contained in the diet.

Secondly, it is the ratio of L.D.L. (low-density lipoprotein) to H.D.L. (high-density lipoprotein) that is important, and not simply the total amount of cholesterol in the diet that is related to the risk of heart disease. One should have a low intake of L.D.L., the "bad" cholesterol, and high intake of H.D.L., the "good" cholesterol.

Thirdly, if cholesterol of any type is so bad for us, why does our body make so much of it? The reason is, of course, that it is a vital substance, the building material of many structural cell components, and the precursor molecule for production of steroid hormones (estrogen, testosterone, adrenaline, etc.)

FUNCTIONS OF E.F.A.S

The following list includes scientifically proven functions of essential fatty acids:

❀ increase energy production by helping the body to obtain more oxygen
❀ improve energy levels and stamina
❀ increase strength and endurance
❀ speed up recovery from fatigue
❀ increase metabolic rate
❀ balance blood-sugar levels
❀ increase excess water loss via the kidneys
❀ prevent food cravings
❀ improve circulation
❀ balance hormones and prostaglandins
❀ fight infection
❀ prevent abnormal growths
❀ improve the skin
❀ reduce stress and anxiety
❀ elevate mood

Since the effectiveness of essential oils is so easily destroyed it is important to have a fresh daily source.

LEFT *The risk of heart disease increases as we get older, but low fat doesn't mean no fat – the body needs essential fatty acids.*

RELATIVE CALORIFIC VALUE OF FOODS

Each gram (about a quarter of an ounce) of fat or oil consumed supplies 9.3Kcals (39Kjoules) of energy. This is around double the calorific value of either protein or carbohydrate, which release 4.0Kcals (16.8Kjoules), and 3.75Kcals (15.8Kjoules) of energy respectively when they are metabolized. This is an additional reason for keeping fats and oils at a low level in our diet.

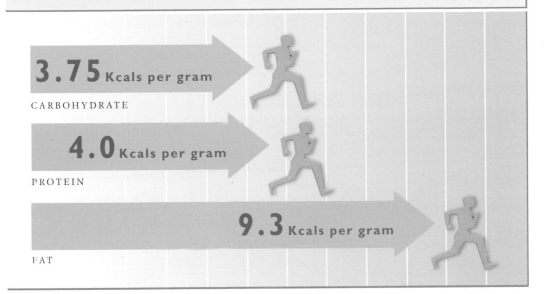

3.75 Kcals per gram

CARBOHYDRATE

4.0 Kcals per gram

PROTEIN

9.3 Kcals per gram

FAT

Fourthly, although high blood cholesterol levels are related to heart disease, there is still extensive heart disease in people who have moderate or low levels. Also, there is little association between high blood cholesterol and death from heart disease in the elderly, or between cholesterol in the diet (from eggs and fatty meat) and blood cholesterol levels. In fact, more than 80 percent of the body's cholesterol comes from that made in the liver, and not from the diet. Patients with heart disease who are instructed to cut down severely on dietary cholesterol and saturated fat, tend to eat massive amounts of carbohydrates. Frequently these are of the refined variety, and are low in manganese, zinc, magnesium, potassium, and chromium, which are the very nutrients needed to nourish a healthy heart. The elevation of insulin levels needed by this high carbohydrate diet may lead to the production of more cholesterol.

It is important to keep H.D.L.s high and reduce damaging L.D.L.s. Mono-unsaturates (in olive oil, groundnuts, and avocados) do this. Polyunsaturates lower both types of cholesterol, but are nevertheless necessary for their essential fatty acid content. A well-balanced diet, such as that recommended in the New Food Pyramid program, optimizes intake of mono-unsaturates and essential fatty acids alike, to fulfill all biochemical functions.

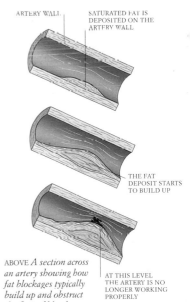

ARTERY WALL

SATURATED FAT IS DEPOSITED ON THE ARTERY WALL

THE FAT DEPOSIT STARTS TO BUILD UP

ABOVE *A section across an artery showing how fat blockages typically build up and obstruct the flow of blood.*

AT THIS LEVEL THE ARTERY IS NO LONGER WORKING PROPERLY

Understanding Proteins

PROTEINS ARE *made up of basic units called amino acids. They are vital for growth and the repair and maintenance of body tissue. Amino acids are also the basis of many hormones, enzymes, antibodies, and neurotransmitters, and they are carriers of fats, oxygen, and other substances within the blood.*

Protein does not need to be consumed in excessive amounts to fulfill its functions. If protein is eaten in excess of body requirements, it cannot be stored by the body in this form (apart from a minute pool of amino acids in each body cell), and has to be converted to carbohydrate or fat. This process is carried out by the liver and requires the removal of nitrogenous

BELOW *Without protein we would never grow, and our bodily tissues would not be renewed.*

material that would otherwise become toxic to the system. In such circumstances the liver and the kidneys have to work hard to remove waste products and are under stress.

What is left of the amino acids at this stage is a carbohydrate-like skeleton that, in normal circumstances, is metabolized to produce energy. If this energy is not used it is converted to fat for storage; consequently, excess protein can cause body fat to build up. Moreover, excess protein makes the body tissues very acidic, and the body has to release calcium and other mineral salts from the skeleton to buffer this excess acidity. Diets high in protein are therefore likely to be one of the possible causes of osteoporosis and other conditions affecting the skeleton.

As with fats, both the quantity and the quality of protein we eat is important. British government recommendations suggest we obtain around 15 percent of our total calorie intake from protein; the New Pyramid program recommends a

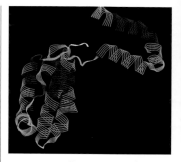

ABOVE *Proteins consist of amino acids, of which several are essential to all human beings.*

more balanced 30 percent. No further governmental advice is given on the types or quality of protein that are best to eat. However, information along these lines is vital to a successful health-giving diet. In the past animal proteins were regarded as "first-class" proteins simply because each one contains all eight of the essential amino acids, which are easily assimilated. However, as you get older animal protein may become harder to digest. In addition, it is more likely to contain saturated fat, and it may also be carrying antibiotic and hormone residues, unless you eat organic meat and dairy foods.

Plant proteins are a less contaminated form of protein, especially if obtained from a pesticide-free source. However, protein from any one plant source may need to be balanced with other plant proteins to obtain the same range of amino acids as in animal protein. Furthermore, vegetable protein tends to contain additional beneficial complex carbohydrates, as in the case of beans and lentils, and is less acid-forming than fish, meat, and some dairy products.

However, although fish and lean meat are high acid-forming foods, they were a major part of our ancestral diet, and are undeniably well suited to our digestive capabilities and metabolism. Fish, especially, is important for its content of D.H.A. and E.P.A. fatty acids. As a general guide, it is best to eat fish in preference to meat; to limit lean meat to three times a week; and to restrict dairy foods (since these are fairly new in evolutionary terms) to a very small amount, say ⅔ cup (150ml) of milk or 1 ounce (27g) cheese, or one small pot of (live) yogurt daily, or slightly larger amounts but less frequently. It is a complete myth to insist that milk and cheese are an essential part of the diet because of their calcium content:

❖ Vegans do not suffer more than dairy-food eaters from calcium-deficiency diseases.

❖ Since milk reduces stomach acidity, it may make calcium less readily absorbed (calcium needs an acid environment for its absorption).

❖ Milk proteins (casein etc) are allergenic in susceptible individuals.

❖ Some adults are sensitive to lactose (milk sugar).

❖ You can get all the calcium you need from seeds (especially sesame), tofu, and dark green vegetables.

ESSENTIAL AMINO ACIDS

Isoleucine	Tryptophan
Leucine	Valine
Lysine	Arginine*
Methionine	Histidine*
Phenylalanine	Taurine*
Threonine	

*Conditionally essential

It is very easy to achieve adequate protein intake whether you are a meat-eater, a vegetarian, or a vegan, since many vegetables, such as runner beans, peas, corn, and broccoli supply good levels of protein. Recent findings indicate that protein high in the essential amino acid methionine may be problematical. Excess methionine produces a substance called homocysteine, which is now known to cause arterial damage leading to cardiovascular disease. Meat, dairy food, and fish are all high in methionine; good quality plant protein has more moderate levels. Vitamins B_6, B_{12}, and folic acid have been shown to protect against homocysteine production.

Meat-eaters should therefore consider eating vegetable protein for three or four days a week to help neutralize excess tissue acidity and prevent loss of calcium and other minerals, maximize levels of B vitamins, and prevent the buildup of damaging homocysteine.

ALL THE AMINO ACIDS OF MEAT CAN BE FOUND IN VEGETABLES, PULSES AND GRAINS

HEAVY MEAT EATING PRODUCES ACIDITY IN BODY TISSUE

RIGHT *Meat eaters often assume that vegetarians lack quality proteins, but this is a myth.*

Understanding Carbohydrate, Fiber, and Water

CARBOHYDRATE IS *the main fuel for the body, responsible for supplying it with energy. Fiber controls blood-sugar levels and regulates bowel movements. Drinking water replenishes the large amounts lost daily through the skin, lungs, gut, and urine.*

CARBOHYDRATE

Unlike fats and proteins, carbohydrate has no other function in the body than to supply it with energy, apart from a small amount of dietary carbohydrate that is vital for the structural basis of D.N.A. and other important molecules. Carbohydrate exists in nature, in two main forms: the "sugars" and the "starches". The first of these are made up of simple monosaccharide sugars, such as glucose and fructose (fruit sugar), and disaccharide sugars such as sucrose ("sugar"), maltose (malt) from germinating grain, and lactose from milk. Starches, on the other hand, are made up of polysaccharides, which are long chains of simple sugars, usually predominantly glucose.

Another natural polysaccharide is cellulose, obtained from plant cell walls (and, therefore, from all fresh vegetables and fruit), and from cereal husks, and seed coats (and, therefore, from brown rice, whole oats, beans, and seeds). Since humans do not possess a cellulose-degrading enzyme, cellulose becomes the "fiber" in your diet.

Starchy vegetables (potatoes, parsnips, corn, peas, broad beans) and grains (whole wheat, rye, oats, barley, rice, millet, maize) are the best sources of starch. If you are gluten-sensitive, you can choose from rice, corn, millet, tapioca, amaranth, buckwheat, and quinoa, which are all gluten-free.

Natural monosaccharide sugars (glucose and fructose), and disaccharide sugars (sucrose, maltose,

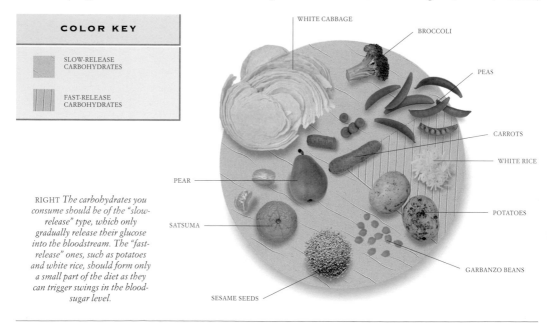

COLOR KEY

SLOW-RELEASE CARBOHYDRATES

FAST-RELEASE CARBOHYDRATES

WHITE CABBAGE

BROCCOLI

PEAS

CARROTS

WHITE RICE

PEAR

POTATOES

SATSUMA

GARBANZO BEANS

SESAME SEEDS

RIGHT *The carbohydrates you consume should be of the "slow-release" type, which only gradually release their glucose into the bloodstream. The "fast-release" ones, such as potatoes and white rice, should form only a small part of the diet as they can trigger swings in the blood-sugar level.*

and lactose), are obtained from sweet vegetables like carrots and beets, fruit, honey, malt, milk, sugar cane, sugar beet, and molasses. Other sweet foods in our diet come, predominantly, from sucrose-containing refined foods, such as cakes, cookies, pastry, candies, chocolate, puddings, custards, and alcohol; you need to be ruthless in cutting these from your diet.

Substances called glycosinolates are produced when "sugar" intake is high; the excess glucose reacts with protein and cells in the blood, to produce "advanced glycation end products" – A.G.E. proteins. These are related to biological aging (at least in animals) and interfere with metabolism by increasing the level of toxic substances associated with damage to the endocrine, immune, and nervous systems.

Generally, foods containing some "sugar" release glucose easily and quickly into the bloodstream, whereas starches, especially when eaten as vegetables, fruit, and wholegrains, take much longer to digest, releasing their glucose a little at a time. This slow-release mechanism works to prevent drastic swings in blood-sugar level. When your blood-sugar level is stable, your energy level is more balanced and you have longer relief from hunger.

Slow-release carbohydrate foods such as vegetables, pulses (legumes), seeds, and fresh fruit should provide about 80 percent of your carbohydrate intake with the remaining 20 percent of your intake provided by carbohydrate-dense foods such as potatoes, wholegrains, bread, pasta, and dried fruit.

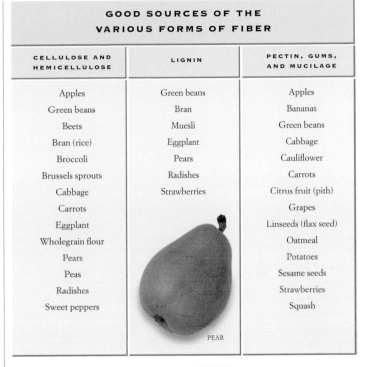

GOOD SOURCES OF THE VARIOUS FORMS OF FIBER

CELLULOSE AND HEMICELLULOSE	LIGNIN	PECTIN, GUMS, AND MUCILAGE
Apples	Green beans	Apples
Green beans	Bran	Bananas
Beets	Muesli	Green beans
Bran (rice)	Eggplant	Cabbage
Broccoli	Pears	Cauliflower
Brussels sprouts	Radishes	Carrots
Cabbage	Strawberries	Citrus fruit (pith)
Carrots		Grapes
Eggplant		Linseeds (flax seed)
Wholegrain flour		Oatmeal
Pears		Potatoes
Peas		Sesame seeds
Radishes		Strawberries
Sweet peppers		Squash

PEAR

FIBER

If your diet includes plenty of fresh fruit, vegetables, pulses (legumes), seeds, nuts, and wholegrains, you will automatically be consuming sufficient fiber in the form of cellulose, hemicellulose, lignin, pectins, gums, and mucilage. Fibrous foods help to reduce the appetite, as well as helping to control blood-sugar levels by allowing sugar to be released from food more slowly. A high-fiber diet will prevent constipation and severe bowel problems, encourage the efficient elimination of waste products, and aid the absorption and excretion of excess cholesterol.

The most healthful fiber is found, in descending order of importance, in apples, rice bran, beets, peas, brown rice, and oats.

WATER

Water is not depicted in the New Pyramid program diagram, but no one would deny that it is vital for life. Despite the fact that water has no calorific value, it plays an important part in the process of eliminating toxic substances from the body. Approximately 6 cups (1.5 liters) of water are lost daily through the skin, lungs, gut, and as urine. However, when carbohydrates are metabolized, about 1¼ cups (0.4 liters) per day of water is made available to the body.

To replace the difference between that lost and that gained ("metabolic" water), we need to drink just over 4 cups (1 liter) of water (or diluted fruit juice and herb and fruit teas) a day.

Vitamins and Minerals

VITAMINS AND MINERALS *are frequently referred to as the "micronutrients" in contrast to fats, protein, and carbohydrates, which are called the "macronutrients". The reason for this is related to the amounts of each nutrient needed by the body. Macronutrients are required in weights that are easily measured by ordinary kitchen scales; despite being essential, micronutrients are only required in very small amounts. There are excellent sources of vitamins and minerals in both plant and animal foods.*

It is a myth to say that vegetarians and vegans cannot obtain all the essential nutrients from their diet. Where quantities of a particular nutrient are low in vegetable foods, absorption rates are enhanced in vegetarians and vegans. Nevertheless, if the diet is not optimum, the digestive system of a meat-eater or vegan alike may function poorly, reducing absorption of micronutrients.

VITAMINS

Vitamins are not structural components of the body, unlike some minerals (such as calcium in the bones), but they have a biochemical function in that they are needed, in conjunction with enzymes, to allow chemical reactions within the cell to proceed. For example, the transport of glucose from the blood into the cells of the body depends upon the presence of vitamins B_3 and B_6, and the actual breakdown of glucose within the cells into energy requires vitamins B_1, B_2, B_3, B_5, and C.

In addition to helping with the release of energy from nutrients within the body, vitamins are needed for a host of other essential functions to be performed effectively: to balance hormone levels, to boost the immune system, to strengthen the skin and connective tissue, to protect the arteries, to assist brain function, and for the transmission of nervous impulses.

MEASUREMENTS

Most vitamins and minerals are measured by weight:

microgram = mcg
milligram (or 1,000mcg) = mg
gram (or 1,000mg) = g

IU (International units) is a measurement system for vitamins A, D, and E. Many supplements are still sold in IUs, but most scientists prefer to measure vitamins by weight:

I iu vitamin A = 0.3mcg
I iu vitamin D = 0.025mcg
I iu vitamin E = 0.7mcg

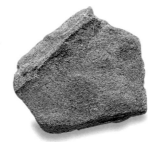

ABOVE *Copper, which can be found in seafood and in nuts, plays an important role in the production of hormones.*

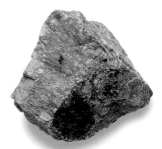

ABOVE *Bone formation and the production of red blood cells are not possible without phosphorus, which is found in meat, fish, and wholegrains.*

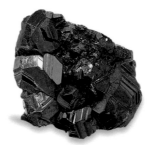

LEFT *Iron is a constituent of hemoglobin, which carries oxygen in the bloodstream.*

Vitamins can be divided into two categories: the water-soluble vitamins, which are not stored in the body and which must therefore be taken daily; and the fat-soluble vitamins, which can be stored in larger amounts. The table on pages 34-35 illustrates the variety of their actions within the body and summarizes the best food sources for obtaining them.

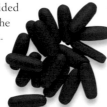

ABOVE *Some vitamin pills also contain iron. Iron is important for the correct functioning of the blood.*

MINERALS

The essential minerals in food go to make up only around 4 percent of your body tissues. Most of this is composed of the "macrominerals" – calcium, magnesium, phosphorus, sodium, chloride, and potassium. These are largely involved with the structural part of the skeleton and the teeth, and as electrolytic salts in the blood and tissue fluids. Correct nutrition is vital to obtain sufficient amounts of these within the body because they are not as abundant as the "macronutrients". There are also fourteen or so "microminerals", commonly called "trace elements" because they are only needed in trace amounts in the body and are found in very tiny amounts in foods. It is even more crucial to insure that this latter group of nutrients is adequately supplied by the diet in order to avoid deficiency.

Minerals, like vitamins, are essential for just about every process in the body. However, unlike vitamins, some minerals become incorporated into body structures, for example calcium, magnesium, and phosphorus, which are found in the bones. Others are similar to vitamins in taking an essential role in metabolism, acting as coenzymes, for example magnesium, zinc, and some copper. However, other minerals have very specific functions, such as iron, which has a very important role as part of the structure of hemoglobin molecules.

As with the vitamins, many minerals are co-workers, this means that the absence of one mineral severely disrupts the functions of other minerals, and ultimately leads to the disruption of the body's metabolism. The table of minerals and their functions on pages 36–37 shows how they work together and lists suitable food sources – it is generally considered preferable to obtain both minerals and vitamins as a part of your regular diet.

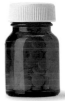

ABOVE *Vitamins can be taken as pills, especially when large doses are required.*

MINERALS AND THE BODY

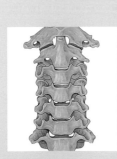

Bones require several minerals. Calcium, phosphorus, boron, fluorine, magnesium, manganese, and silicon are all essential.

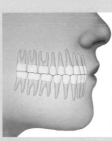

Teeth, like bones, need calcium, phosphorus, and fluorine. Most calcium absorbed in the diet goes to the teeth and bones.

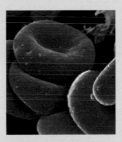

The production of red blood cells requires phosphorus and copper, while iron is the central element of hemoglobin.

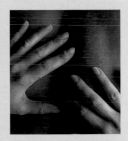

The state of the skin is often a sign of how healthy the body's cells are overall. They depend on supplies of zinc, magnesium, iron, and other minerals.

Guide to Vitamins and Minerals

THE TABLES ON *the following pages provide a comprehensive guide to vitamins, minerals, and trace elements. They outline the functions performed by specific vitamins and minerals, and explain, in every case, the best food sources. As long as you obtain your vitamins and minerals from the good wholesome food sources in a balanced diet there is no need to worry about "overdosing".*

GUIDE TO VITAMINS

Vitamin A • Retinol and betacarotene
Essential for normal vision (especially night vision), skin, mucous membranes of the respiratory, digestive and urinary tracts, growth of bones and tissues, reproduction and immunity. It is an antioxidant and fat-soluble.
BEST FOOD SOURCES: Retinol – liver, fish-liver oils. Betacarotene – carrots and green leafy vegetables. Generally, there is a higher betacarotene content in intensely colored vegetables.

Vitamin B₁ • Thiamine
Essential for releasing energy from carbohydrates, and for the integrity of the nervous system. It is water-soluble.
BEST FOOD SOURCES: wholegrains, seeds, beans, and nuts.

Vitamin B₂ • Riboflavin
Essential for metabolizing carbohydrates, fats, and proteins. It is especially important in assisting many enzymes in the liver to enable the efficient removal of toxins. This vitamin is water-soluble.
BEST FOOD SOURCES: kidney, liver, fish, milk, wheatgerm, broccoli, and green leafy vegetables.

Vitamin B₃ • Niacin, Niacinamide/Nicotinamide
Essential for releasing energy from carbohydrates, and the metabolism of proteins, fats, and polyunsaturated fatty acids. Additionally, it is vital for the formation of red blood cells and steroid hormones. It is water-soluble.
BEST FOOD SOURCES: liver, poultry, fish, meat, groundnuts, wholegrains, eggs, and milk.

Vitamin B₅ • Pantothenic Acid
Essential for making glycogen (energy stores) and fatty acids in the body. Also required for making neurotransmitter chemicals (chemicals that transfer nerve impulses), and for the steroid hormones (sex hormones) testosterone and estrogen. It is water-soluble.
BEST FOOD SOURCES: groundnuts, liver, kidney, egg yolks, fish, wholegrains, beans, and nuts.

Vitamin B₆ • Pyridoxine, Pyridoxal-5-Phosphate
Essential for protein and amino acid metabolism, for promoting a healthy cardiovascular system, and in producing hemoglobin (the oxygen-carrying pigment in blood). It is water-soluble.
BEST FOOD SOURCES: wheatgerm, seeds, chicken, lamb, fish, eggs, bananas, avocados, soybeans, walnuts, and oats.

Folate • Folic acid, Folacin
Essential for transporting coenzymes needed for amino acid metabolism in the body. Especially needed by children during growth, and where cell turnover is rapid such as in red blood cells. It is vital for of a growing fetus; water-soluble.
BEST FOOD SOURCES: wheatgerm, fresh dark green leafy vegetables (especially spinach), beans, egg yolks, asparagus, whole wheat, lamb's liver, and salmon.

RIGHT *Green leafy vegetables are one of the best sources of vitamin B₂.*

Vitamin B₁₂ • Cyanocobalamin
Essential for efficient working of every cell in the body, especially those cells that undergo rapid turnover, such as red blood cells, the gut lining, and blood vessels. It is essential for the proper functioning of the nervous system. It is water-soluble.
BEST FOOD SOURCES: liver, oysters, poultry, fish, eggs, fermented foods such as miso (fermented soybean paste), and tempeh (fermented whole soybeans).

Biotin
Essential for helping enzymes in the manufacture of glycogen and fatty acids in the body, and in the production of prostaglandins (compounds involved with normal immune function). It is essential for normal growth and development of the skin, hair, nerves, and bone marrow. It is water-soluble.
BEST FOOD SOURCES: liver, sardines, egg yolks, soy, wholegrains, nuts, and beans.

Vitamin C • Ascorbate, Ascorbic acid
Essential for formation of collagen, skin integrity, tissue repair, effective action of white cells and antibodies, and the immune system in general. Acts as an antioxidant, and helps to normalize blood cholesterol levels. Water-soluable.
BEST FOOD SOURCES: guava, Brussels sprouts, cranberries, blackcurrants, kiwi fruit, papaw, mango, broccoli, cauliflower, tomatoes, strawberries, and citrus fruit.

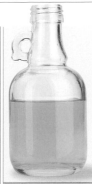

LEFT *Olive oil is an excellent source of vitamin E – essential for fighting the damaging effects of free radicals.*

Vitamin D • Cholecalciferol
Essential for bone growth and balancing mineral levels within the body. It is needed for the proper absorption of calcium and phosphorus from the intestines. Sunlight on the skin will produce vitamin D. Like vitamin A, it is fat-soluble.
BEST FOOD SOURCES: fish-liver oils, fortified milk, and fatty fish. Unlikely to be deficient in the diet.

OTHER NUTRIENTS RELATED TO VITAMINS

Choline • Phosphatidyl choline
Essential as a neurotransmitter in the brain and nervous system, and as a "fat mobilizer" in the liver.
BEST FOOD SOURCES: soy lecithin, egg yolks, liver, fish, and wholegrains. The body can make it from other nutrients.

Inositol
Essential for the normal metabolism of calcium and insulin. May also be involved in fatty acid metabolism.
BEST FOOD SOURCES: soy lecithin, egg yolks, liver, fish, citrus fruit (except lemons), milk, nuts, and wholegrains. The body can make it from other nutrients.

RIGHT *Eggs are a good source of choline, needed for the production of neurotransmitters.*

Vitamin E • Tocopherol
Essential as an antioxidant for protecting essential fatty acids (and, therefore, cell membranes and blood vessels) from oxidation damage due to free-radical activity. Also involved in the reproductive system. It is fat-soluble.
BEST FOOD SOURCES: wheatgerm oil, wheatgerm, soybean oil, olive oil, egg yolk, liver, and nuts (especially almonds and walnuts).

Coenzyme Q10 • Ubiquinone
Essential for all energy production within the cell as part of the electron transport system, immunity, heart function, and as an antioxidant.
BEST FOOD SOURCES: heart and other organ meats, meat, egg yolk, milk fat, wheatgerm, and wholegrains.

Carnitine
Helps in the carriage of fats and fatty acids in the blood.
BEST FOOD SOURCES: lamb, chicken, and animal foods in general. Can be made in the body.

Vitamin K • Phylloquinone
Essential for blood clotting, especially in newborn babies. It is fat-soluble.
BEST FOOD SOURCES: raw cauliflower, and green leafy vegetables. It is also made by the bacteria in the gut.

BELOW *Raw cauliflower is rich in vitamin K, necessary for efficient blood clotting.*

Bioflavonoids
There are over 500 different bioflavonoid compounds and they are almost all substances needed by plants for photosynthesis. They increase the potency of antioxidants and maintain cell membranes, especially those lining blood vessels, and collagen.
BEST FOOD SOURCES: white rind of citrus fruit, vegetables, buckwheat, and honey.

Pyrroloquinoline quinone • P.Q.Q.
Involved in collagen metabolism.
BEST FOOD SOURCE: fresh citrus fruit.

RIGHT *P.Q.Q., found in citrus fruit, is vital for the manufacture of collagen.*

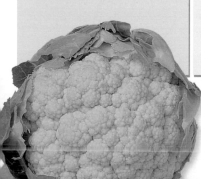

THE MICROMINERALS (TRACE ELEMENTS)

Boron
Essential for the manufacture of many hormones, formation of bone, balance of estrogen.
BEST FOOD SOURCES: alfalfa, cabbage, lettuce, peas, soybeans, almonds, hazelnuts, apples, prunes, raisins, and dates.

Cobalt
Forms an essential part of vitamin B12.
BEST FOOD SOURCES: liver, kidney, oyster, meat, fish, and sea vegetables.

LEFT *The beneficial amounts of copper contained in cashews help to maintain the production of blood cells.*

Chromium
Essential for efficient glucose metabolism (as Glucose Tolerance Factor), insulin production, fatty acid metabolism, and protein metabolism.
BEST FOOD SOURCES: wholegrains, shellfish, liver, pulses (legumes), black pepper, and molasses.

Iodine
Forms part of thyroxine, the thyroid hormone, which regulates energy production in the body.
BEST FOOD SOURCES: haddock, mackerel, cod, live yogurt, seaweed, and iodized salt.

Manganese
Essential for normal formation of bone and cartilage, and for control of glucose metabolism. It is also part of the antioxidant superoxide dismutase, which helps prevent free radical damage.
BEST FOOD SOURCES: wholegrains, rice bran, wheatgerm, black tea, nuts, ginger, and cloves.

Molybdenum
Forms part of at least three enzyme systems, and is an important antioxidant.
BEST FOOD SOURCES: wholegrains, pulses (legumes), buckwheat, wheatgerm, liver, and sunflower seeds.

Copper
Essential for many enzymes, especially those controlling normal production of blood cells and hormones. Too much copper will depress zinc levels.
BEST FOOD SOURCES: organ meat, seafood, cherries, nuts (especially cashews), olives, and cocoa.

Fluorine
Important for bone and tooth structure, and may help to prevent heart disease.
BEST FOOD SOURCES: seafood, meat, and tea.

RIGHT *Seafood has a high fluorine content.*

Iron
Iron is the central element in the oxygen-carrying blood pigment hemoglobin.
BEST FOOD SOURCES: cockles, molasses, cocoa, liver, meats, wheatgerm, clams, prunes, seaweed, and spinach.
Note: animal sources of iron are absorbed better than vegetable forms. Absorption of iron is enhanced by taking vitamin C at the same meal.

Selenium
Essential for many key enzymes in the body. It is an antioxidant, which neutralizes free radicals.
BEST FOOD SOURCES: Brazil nuts, molasses, cashews, soybeans, tuna, seafood, meat, and wholegrains. Also present in many vegetables, but the amount is dependent upon the presence of selenium in the soil.

Nickel
Essential for normal growth.
BEST FOOD SOURCES: widely distributed in fruit and vegetables. Tiny amounts transfer from stainless steel pans.

Vanadium
Vanadium is an interesting mineral. The latest research indicates its involvement in the sodium/potassium pump mechanism that is present in all cells, and may implicate the mineral in instances where there is an inability to lose weight.
BEST FOOD SOURCES: black pepper, soy oil, corn oil, olive oil, olives.

Silicon

Involved in normal bone growth, and is needed for healthy skin, hair, and membranes.
BEST FOOD SOURCES: wholegrains and seaweed.

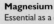

LEFT *Seaweed contains silicon, important for healthy skin and hair.*

Zinc

Essential for metabolism, as zinc forms part of many enzymes involved in cell growth, immunity, production of testosterone (the male hormone), sperm formation, and libido. Required for normal production of stomach acid.
BEST FOOD SOURCES: seafood (especially oysters), popcorn, pumpkin seeds, sesame seeds, fish, wheatgerm, meat, and eggs.

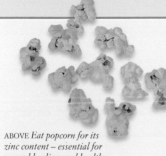

ABOVE *Eat popcorn for its zinc content – essential for wound healing, and healthy growth and repair of cells.*

Other minerals found in the human body include cadmium, germanium, tin, aluminium, arsenic, barium, bromine, gold, lead, mercury, and strontium. It is not yet clear whether these are actually required by the body in the minute amounts in which they are found, or whether they are in fact toxic trace impurities from the environment.

THE MACROMINERALS

Calcium

Essential for bones and teeth, where most dietary calcium is found. The remainder moves in and out of cells allowing conduction of impulses between nerves, and the contraction of muscles. Excess calcium depresses magnesium levels.
BEST FOOD SOURCES: cooked bones (as in canned fish), whitebait, homemade fish stock, tofu, sesame seeds, and dairy products.

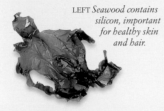

ABOVE *Sesame seeds are an excellent source of immune-boosting calcium and magnesium.*

Sodium

One of the body's electrolytes, which are electrically charged atoms (together with potassium and chloride), performing essential functions in the cells. Sodium is the main cation (positively charged electrolyte) in the extra-cellular fluid. There is too much sodium in most people's diet. Even if you never use convenience foods, and never add common salt to your food, you will still obtain sufficent sodium from vegetables.

Potassium

The third of the body's electrolytes. It is the main cation (positively charged electrolyte) within the cells. It interacts with sodium and chloride in maintaining an optimum environment in and around each body cell.
BEST FOOD SOURCES: tomato paste, dried apricots, figs, bananas, pumpkin seeds, almonds, soybeans, potatoes (especially baked), green leafy vegetables, fish, avocados, beans, fruit, and vegetables.

Magnesium

Essential as a component of bone, and in general metabolism where it is part of over 300 enzymes. It is also needed for the oxidation of glycogen for energy, muscle relaxation, and in the formation of new proteins within each cell. Excess magnesium depresses calcium levels.
BEST FOOD SOURCES: wholegrains, lima beans, taco shells, black-eyed peas, fish, seeds, wheatgerm, dried apricots, dark green vegetables, soybeans, buckwheat.

Phosphorus

Essential for bone formation and production of red blood cells. A vital part of A.T.P. (Adenosine Tri-Phosphate), which is the chemical energy store in every cell of the body, and D.N.A.
BEST FOOD SOURCES: meats, fish, and wholegrains.

Chloride

Another of the body's electrolytes. It is the main anion (negatively charged electrolyte) in the extra-cellular fluid. Along with sodium, most diets contain too much chloride, as common salt (sodium chloride). A healthy, balanced diet, such as the New Pyramid program, will contain sufficient chloride.

BELOW *Potassium is needed for a healthy nervous system; potatoes and green leafy vegetables are abundant sources of this mineral.*

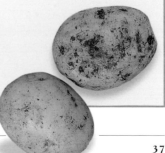

Proper Use of Supplements

THERE IS A VAST *range of nutritional supplements on the market, making it very difficult for the layperson to choose. As a general precaution, you would be best advised to self-prescribe only the multiformulas that cover a broad spectrum of nutrients in one capsule or tablet, since taking isolated nutrient supplements can have a disastrous effect on the metabolism.*

While there are some excellent, high-quality products on the market, some are nearly useless. Generally, you get what you pay for. To get the best out of your supplement regime, consider a few basic principles. These relate to the variability in the absorption rate of different nutrients. Additionally, almost all nutrients have other nutrients that help their absorption (synergists), and some that hinder it (antagonists). Absorption rates can be enhanced by following these simple guidelines.

HOW TO IMPROVE NUTRIENT ABSORPTION

❋ Keep alcohol and supplements separate – alcohol will leach these supplements immediately. The one exception is vitamin C, which can help counterbalance the effects of alcohol.

❋ Avoid drinking tea and coffee at meal times, or within one hour either side of taking your supplement – these beverages have a leaching effect on nutrients.

❋ Do not smoke for at least 30 minutes either side of a meal or taking supplements – the chemicals in tobacco smoke have a leaching effect on nutrients and use up antioxidants in the process.

❋ Eat slowly – stressful activities (like eating too fast) can impair digestion and prevent absorption.

❋ Fat-soluble vitamins are best taken with meals that contain some fat – this will help "escort" them into the body.

❋ Foods high in B-complex vitamins (e.g. cereals), and vitamin B-complex supplements are best taken early in the day, since they kick-start the metabolism.

❋ Calming supplements like magnesium, calcium, and zinc are best taken half an hour or so before bedtime.

❋ Take a combined multiformula supplement in the morning, but an hour after breakfast cereal.

❋ Never take supplements, especially those containing minerals, on an empty stomach; they may bring on nausea. Amino acids and some probiotics are an exception to this rule.

❋ Never take "single" supplements except under the guidance of a nutritional therapist.

❋ Begin and stop taking supplements gradually to give your body time to adjust.

❋ Eat adequate levels of a good variety of fiber, and some live yogurt (or a probiotic supplement) to keep the intestines healthy and therefore enhance absorption rates.

BELOW *Supplementary vitamins should not be taken within an hour of drinking tea or coffee.*

HOW TO GET THE BEST USE FROM SUPPLEMENTS

Get the best out of your supplement by taking it at the appropriate time and with "helpers"
in supplement form or obtained from food if possible, which will have a beneficial effect on its absorption.

SUPPLEMENT	WHEN TO TAKE	HELPERS	HINDERERS
Vitamin A	With fatty food	Zinc, vitamins E and C	Lack of bile
Vitamin D	With fatty food	Calcium, phosphorus, vitamins E and C, sunlight	Lack of bile
Vitamin E	With fatty food	Selenium, vitamin C	Ferric iron, fried food
Vitamin B1	Early in day	Vitamin B-complex, manganese	Alcohol, stress, antibiotics, cooking
Vitamin B2	Early in day	Vitamin B-complex	Alcohol, stress, antibiotics, tobacco, cooking
Vitamin B3	Early in day	Vitamin B-complex	Alcohol, stress, antibiotics, cooking
Vitamin B5	Early in day	Vitamin B-complex, biotin, folic acid	Stress, antibiotics, cooking
Vitamin B6	Early in day	Magnesium, zinc, Vitamin B-complex	Alcohol, stress, antibiotics, cooking
Vitamin B12	Early in day	Calcium, vitamin B-complex, folic acid	Alcohol, stress, antibiotics, cooking, internal parasites
Folic Acid	Early in day	Vitamin C, B-complex	Alcohol, stress, antibiotics
Biotin	Early in day	Vitamin B-complex	Stress, avidin in raw egg white, antibiotics
Choline	Early in day	Vitamin B5	Alcohol, stress, antibiotics
Inositol	Early in day	Choline	Alcohol, stress, antibiotics
Vitamin C	Between meals	Hydrochloric acid (HCl)	Heavy metals, cooking
Calcium	With protein food or at bedtime	Magnesium, vitamin D, HCl	Tea, coffee, smoking, phytic acid
Magnesium	With protein food or at bedtime	Calcium, vitamin B6, vitamin D, HCl	Tea, coffee, smoking, alcohol, excess iron
Iron	With any food	Vitamin C, HCl	Tea, coffee, smoking, oxalic & phytic acids
Zinc	With food or at bedtime	Vitamin B6 and vitamin C, HCl	Phytic acid, lead, copper, coffee, alcohol, excess iron
Manganese	With protein food	Vitamin C, HCl	High dosage zinc, tea, coffee, smoking, iron
Selenium	With food	Vitamin E, HCl	Mercury, tea, coffee, smoking, excess vitamin C, excess iron
Chromium	With protein food	Vitamin B3, HCl	Tea, coffee, smoking, iron
Iodine	With protein food	Manganese	Tea, coffee, smoking
Molybdenum	With any food	Vitamin B-complex	Tea, coffee, smoking

Antioxidants and Free Radicals

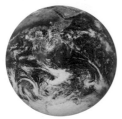

DURING THE *last few years or so, research has confirmed that many of the common diseases and ailments of the Western world (cardiovascular disease, diabetes, cataracts, high blood pressure, infertility, gum disease, respiratory infections, rheumatoid arthritis, Alzheimer's disease, some cancers, and even mental illness) are associated with oxidation and tissue deficiency and low dietary levels of compounds called "antioxidants". Oxidation is a natural occurrence in the world of chemistry and biology.*

Life could not exist without the presence of oxygen; it is the basis of all plant and animal life on earth. Without it we could not release the energy from our food, and without energy the body can do nothing. Furthermore, scavenger cells in our immune system use some of the products of oxidation as weapons against invading micro-organisms. Although it is obviously biologically necessary, oxidation is damaging to whatever is oxidized, but our bodies are forced to risk the damage to obtain the energy they need .

Because oxygen is chemically a very reactive element it can be highly dangerous if not regulated, producing too many "oxidized" molecules inside the body, and creating havoc. During all normal biochemical reactions, oxygen reacts readily to "oxidize" other molecules in its vicinity. If there is nothing available to control this, a cascade of reactions can occur in which the oxidized molecules, "free radicals", become unstable. An army of antioxidant substances keeps any damage to a minimum.

WHAT ARE ANTIOXIDANTS?

Antioxidants are substances that retard or prevent deterioration, damage, or destruction caused by oxidation. Fortunately, the body has a plethora of antioxidants for damage limitation. A family of antioxidant enzymes are provided in

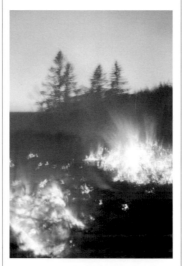

ABOVE *Free radicals are produced wherever combustion occurs, and are therefore present in the environment. They can cause cellular damage unless combatted by antioxidants in the diet.*

healthy tissue, together with substances like cysteine and glutathione. Blood constituents, like the iron-containing transferrin, also act to prevent the production of oxidative-damaging molecules.

In addition to these, many everyday foods – particularly fruit, vegetables, seeds, nuts, and wholegrains – contain a host of antioxidant nutrients that have the power to augment the body's natural antioxidant capacity. Vitamin A, in the form of betacarotene (found in orange and dark green fruit and vegetables), vitamin C (found in fruit and vegetables), vitamin E (found in cereals and seeds), selenium and zinc (found in nuts, seeds, and seafood) are all excellent sources of antioxidants.

Under normal circumstances, when cells utilize oxygen and nutrients to make A.T.P. (the basic energy molecule), the free radicals generated are removed by the system of antioxidant enzymes and nutrients. If there are plentiful amounts of high-energy molecules, essential nutrients, water, and

RIGHT *Pollution is one of the greatest causes of free radicals at a level at which the body cannot cope.*

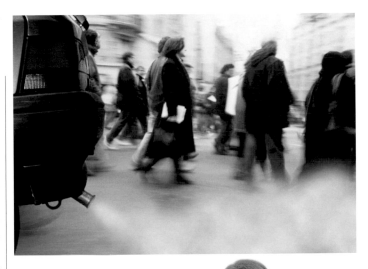

antioxidant enzymes, cell damage is minimized. However, if any of these components are missing, cell damage, aging, and disease follow. The body is forced to employ antioxident nutrients to mop up any free radicals that escape the antioxidant enzymes – these nutrients are very important in fighting a "rearguard" action. A good way to boost enzyme potential is to eat raw foods since the two main digestive enzymes, amylase and protease (which are found in many foods) are destroyed the longer food is cooked.

HOW FREE RADICALS CAUSE DAMAGE

Free radicals are produced wherever combustion occurs, so they will arise from tobacco smoke, exhaust fumes, radiation, and fried or barbecued food. In addition, the "normal" oxidation processes occurring in cells will produce their own range of free radicals. Free radicals can also arise from industrial pollution, too much sun on the skin, infection, excessive exercise, and even stress.

When free radicals are present in excess, this can lead to cellular damage, because important fatty acids and proteins in cell membranes become unstable and their "traffic-directing" effect of balancing the flow of nutrients in and out of the cells becomes ineffective. When the cell membrane is oxidized, it is either hardened so that nutrients cannot get into the cell, or it may be punctured so that the cell collapses as the cell fluid drains out. This process leads to a very familiar sign of aging – wrinkles! The skin cells collapse and harden and this makes the skin sag and look leathery.

Any good diet (such as the New Pyramid program) should encourage the inclusion of foods rich in polyunsaturated oils but it must, at the same time, increase the amount of antioxidant nutrients (beta carotene, vitamins C and E, selenium, etc.) to allow some protection for these oils so that they can be built up appropriately into cellular structures. For example, when stir-frying vegetables in olive oil, the addition of raw garlic (which is full of antioxidants) to the mixture will protect the heated oil.

Years of research have shown that free radicals are the major cause of cell damage in many degenerative diseases. An increase in intake of antioxidant nutrients not only keeps signs of aging at bay, it can also prevent the associated decline into degenerative disease.

OVEREXPOSURE TO THE SUN AND A DIET HIGH IN FRIED FOOD LEAD TO PREMATURE WRINKLES

FREE RADICALS CAN CAUSE INFLAMMATION OF THE JOINTS

LEFT *The signs of aging are visible manifestations of cell damage, often caused by free radicals.*

ANTIOXIDANT ENZYMES

The body creates several enzymes that combat free radicals. When they cannot control the free radicals, possibly because there are too many, then the body is prone to certain identifiable diseases and conditions.

ENZYME	FREE RADICAL ACTED UPON	DISEASES/CONDITIONS RELATED TO EXCESS FREE RADICALS
Superoxide dismutase	Superoxide	Arthritis, bursitis, gout
Catalase	Hydrogen peroxide	Arthritis, bursitis, gout
Glutathione peroxidase	Lipid peroxides and Hydrogen peroxide	Heart disease, liver disease, premature aging, skin cancer, eczema, wrinkling, age spots, dermatitis, psoriasis
Methione reductase	Hydroxyl	Poor recovery from excessive exercise, radiation damage

THE EFFECTS OF AGE AND STRESS

As we have seen, there are several enzymes, made by the body, which control reactive free radicals. The names of some of these enzymes are superoxide dismutase (S.O.D.), catalase, glutathione peroxidase, and methione reductase. Recent research indicates that cellular production of some of these enzymes decreases markedly with age. It is becoming increasingly likely, therefore, that the balance between your body's antioxidant enzyme level (plus your intake of antioxidant nutrients and/or supplements), and your exposure to the huge variety of environmental and internally produced free radicals, is the deciding factor in whether your pathway in life is one of good health.

Each day, many of us are exposed to chemical stress (from various types of environmental pollution), emotional stress (from family, relationships, overwork, financial problems), and physical trauma (from injuries, surgery, and infection). The common denominator in all forms of stress is the overproduction of cell-damaging free radicals.

The major way stress harms us is by weakening our immune system, which becomes overloaded as it tries to process thousands of toxic chemicals. It is imperative, therefore to use stress-reducing techniques to minimize overall stress in our lives. One of the best ways to reduce the amount of free radical damage is to eat foods, such as vegetables, fruit, and whole grains, that contain high levels of antioxidants.

MEDITATION INVOLVES RELAXING PHYSICAL TENSION

BREATHING NATURALLY BECOMES EASIER AND CALMER

RIGHT *By taking you to a deeper level of rest than sleep, meditation is a powerful way of restoring balance in your life.*

ANTIOXIDANT NUTRIENTS

The group of nutrient antioxidants are the body's weapons against free radicals. Some antioxidants are vitamins, such as vitamin A (as betacarotene), vitamin C, and vitamin E. Others are minerals, such as selenium, zinc, and molybdenum. Additional nutrients, such as L-glutathione, N-acetyl cysteine, and Coenzyme Q10, all display antioxidant activity. Yet others, not strictly essential to the body, nevertheless show excellent antioxidant activity. These include such compounds such as anthocyanidins, bioflavonoids, lycopene, pycnogenol, and, possibly, hundreds of other recently identified natural chemicals found in everyday fresh foods. Many herbs also contain excellent ranges of antioxidants.

These substances have a profound effect on aging and the degenerative diseases of the modern age. The protective qualities of antioxidant nutrients increase with concentration of the different nutrients, and many physicians suggest that supplementation of the diet may be necessary to achieve this protection. Supplementing the New Pyramid program with a multi-antioxidant supplement will do no harm and will probably speed up the healing process for many individuals.

RIGHT *Certain herbs and plants, including* Ginkgo biloba, *have excellent antioxidant levels.*

TEN ANTIOXIDANTS FOUND IN FOOD

1 Anthocyanidins, found in berries and grapes, particularly in the skins.

2 Betacarotene, found in orange fruit and vegetables such as apricots and carrots.

3 Bioflavonoids are especially rich in citrus fruit, particularly the white inner rind (hesperidin), buckwheat (rutin), and onions and garlic (quercetin).

4 Curcumin is found in mustard, turmeric, yellow peppers, and corn.

5 Lutein is from the carotene family and is found in many fruits and vegetables, such as spinach and other dark green vegetables. It is extremely heat-stable, it can survive cooking.

6 Lycopene is found in tomatoes.

7 Proanthocyanidins are found in green tea and grape seeds.

8 Pycnogenol occurs in a variety of natural foods, but the most potent source is *Pinus maritima*, a coastal pine tree.

9 Zeazanthin produces the yellow color in corn, and it is also present in spinach, peas, broccoli, and cabbage.

10 Lipoic acid found in yeast and liver

PHYTOCHEMICALS

There is one further group of substances that play a part in nutritional science – "phytochemicals". Phytochemicals are not properly classified as nutrients since our lives do not depend on them in the same way that they depend on proteins, carbohydrates, fats, vitamins, and minerals. Nevertheless, they play an important role in our body's biochemistry. They are closely related

IMPORTANT PHYTOCHEMICALS

This table lists some of the most important phytochemicals and the food sources in which they are found, and describes their roles in healing or in the prevention of disease.

PHYTOCHEMICAL	FOUND IN	IMPORTANT FOR
Allium compounds	Garlic, onions, leeks, chives, and shallots	Proper function of the cardiovascular and immune systems
Capsaicin	Hot peppers	Protecting D.N.A. from damage; pain relief
Chlorophyll and carotenoids	All dark green and orange vegetables, germinated wheatgrains (wheat grass), and seaweed	Healthy red blood cells, protecting against cancer, killing germs, and acting as a wound healer
Coumarins and chorogenic acid	Tomatoes, sweet green peppers, pineapples, strawberries, and carrots	Preventing the formation of cancer-causing nitrosamines in the gut
Genistein	Soybeans	Preventing the growth of tumors; balancing estrogen
Ginkgolides	Ginkgo biloba	Specifically acting as an antioxidant in the brain
Glucosinolate	Brussels sprouts, cabbage, broccoli, and cauliflower	Enhancing detoxification enzyme activity
Ellagic acid	Strawberries, grapes, and raspberries	Neutralizing carcinogens before damage occurs
Isoflavones	Soybeans	Reducing tumor formation
Isothiocyanates and indoles	Broccoli, Brussels sprouts, cabbage, cauliflower, cress, kale, horseradish, mustard, radish, and turnip	Preventing some forms of cancer (especially colon cancer) by deactivating carcinogens
Lentinan	Shiitake mushrooms	Preventing cancer by stimulating the immune system
Lignans	Fibrous vegetables (runner beans, carrots, etc.)	Normalizing estrogen activity.
Phytoestrogens	Soy (tofu and miso), pulses (legumes), citrus fruit, wheat, licorice, alfalfa, fennel, rhubarb, aniseed, and ginseng	Binding xeno-estrogens from the environment; helping with menopausal symptoms, fibroids and other hormone-related problems; reducing the risk of breast cancer
Saponins (diosgenin)	Mexican yams	Stimulating adrenal glands, and the production of progesterone and other sex hormones
Sterols (plant)	Red wine, and chocolate	Preventing oxidation of "bad" (L.D.L.) cholesterol
Sulforaphane (from glucosinolate)	Broccoli, cauliflower, kale, Brussels sprouts, and turnips	Helping to boost the production of anti-cancer enzymes
Tocotrienols	Palm oil, barley oil, rice oil, and rice bran	Helping lower cholesterol

to antioxidants and, in some cases, merge with them. They are the biologically active compounds that are widely found in everyday foods, such as fruit, vegetables, and some grains. So far, well over two hundred of these substances have been isolated and identified, and many appear to have an important effect in regulating the hormonal (endocrine) and immune systems, and hence can help prevent disease.

Building on the knowledge given of how foods work in the body and the particular healing abilities of some of them, the next part of the book will show you how to assess and improve your own situation.

ANTIOXIDANT/PHYTOCHEMICAL FOOD CHOICES

To obtain a good quantity of antioxidants and phytochemicals, choose one item from as many of these groups as possible every day. These are the best vegetables, fruit, grains, seeds, nuts, and so on, to eat as part of your New Pyramid program.

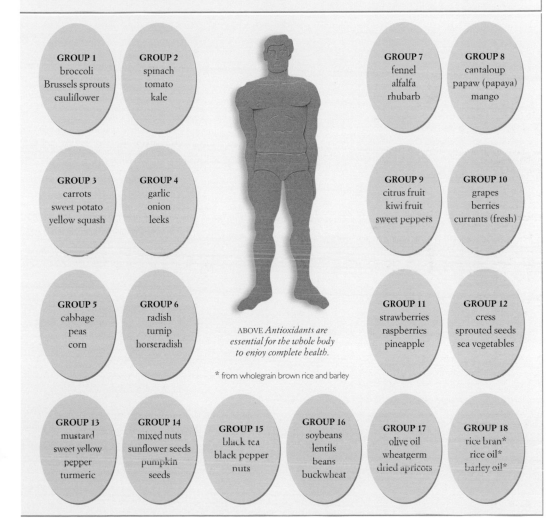

GROUP 1
broccoli
Brussels sprouts
cauliflower

GROUP 2
spinach
tomato
kale

GROUP 7
fennel
alfalfa
rhubarb

GROUP 8
cantaloup
papaw (papaya)
mango

GROUP 3
carrots
sweet potato
yellow squash

GROUP 4
garlic
onion
leeks

GROUP 9
citrus fruit
kiwi fruit
sweet peppers

GROUP 10
grapes
berries
currants (fresh)

GROUP 5
cabbage
peas
corn

GROUP 6
radish
turnip
horseradish

GROUP 11
strawberries
raspberries
pineapple

GROUP 12
cress
sprouted seeds
sea vegetables

ABOVE *Antioxidants are essential for the whole body to enjoy complete health.*

* from wholegrain brown rice and barley

GROUP 13
mustard
sweet yellow
pepper
turmeric

GROUP 14
mixed nuts
sunflower seeds
pumpkin
seeds

GROUP 15
black tea
black pepper
nuts

GROUP 16
soybeans
lentils
beans
buckwheat

GROUP 17
olive oil
wheatgerm
dried apricots

GROUP 18
rice bran*
rice oil*
barley oil*

Where Ailments Originate: The Digestive System

IN TRYING TO *establish advisory nutritional guidelines, we have to recognize that there is no single optimum program that will suit everybody. If we imply that there is, we are paying no attention to what is the basis of nutritional healing – biochemical individuality. We can, however, outline a general program that works well for the majority of people.*

DIGESTION AND ABSORPTION

Digestion is the process whereby ingested food is broken down in the mouth, stomach, duodenum, and ileum by digestive enzymes made in the salivary glands, gastric glands, pancreas, and lining of the ileum. Hydrochloric acid in the stomach is also vital for digestion, especially that of protein.

Minerals and vitamins generally do not need breaking down before they enter the bloodstream. Fiber stays in the digestive tract to help carry away wastes. When any one of these activities is impaired, our ability to digest food declines, beginning the downward spiral to ill-health.

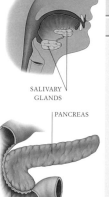

SALIVARY GLANDS

PANCREAS

PANCREAS AND DUODENUM ARE CONNECTED BY A SMALL DUCT

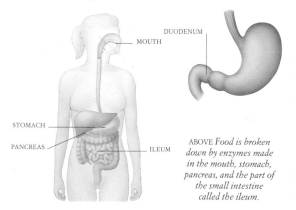

DUODENUM

MOUTH

STOMACH

PANCREAS

ILEUM

ABOVE *Food is broken down by enzymes made in the mouth, stomach, pancreas, and the part of the small intestine called the ileum.*

IS YOUR DIGESTION UP TO SCRATCH?

Give"yes" or "no" answers to the following questions.

❋ Do you have frequent gas in the lower bowel?
❋ Do you suffer from psoriasis, acne, or other skin problems?
❋ Do you have frequent discomfort on the left side of the upper abdomen (around the lower ribs area), or under the left shoulder blade?
❋ Do you suffer frequently from rectal itching?
❋ Do you have a history of asthma, sinus problems, or hay fever?
❋ Do you feel as though your food "sticks" in your stomach (pain or discomfort just behind the lower part of the breast bone)?
❋ Do you feel nauseous frequently?
❋ Do you have either diarrhea or constipation most of the time?
❋ Do you feel bloated often?
❋ Do you have frequent heartburn (reflux into the esophagus), or suffer excessive belching?
❋ Do you have stomach pains or cramps after eating?
❋ Do you have much undigested food in the stools?

SCORING

Score one point for each "yes" answer.

0 – 2 Your digestion seems fine.
3 – 6 You are borderline. Some of your digestive symptoms may be due to stress.
6 and over It is likely that you have a large degree of digestive distress that needs to be dealt with as part of your optimum program, so read on.

THE CAUSES OF POOR DIGESTION

As we get older, the acid in our stomachs is produced less efficiently and can lead to poor chemical and enzymatic digestion of our food, particularly protein. Food may remain in the stomach for longer than normal; it ferments and produces gas (belching) and discomfort. Further problems occur if the pancreas and intestinal lining are functioning poorly and releasing lower levels of their specific enzymes and hormones. As improperly digested food travels through our intestines it irritates the lining and may eventually damage the absorptive layers, resulting in what is commonly called "leaky gut". This leakiness allows fragments of improperly digested foods to pass through the lining into the blood system, and can be the starting point for the development of "intolerance" reactions to foods.

Eating a typical Western diet for several years encourages the wrong type of bacteria to proliferate in the large intestine, causing putrefaction of partially digested food and wastes. Metabolic wastes from these micro-organisms become toxic. They can either set up localized irritation and infection (flatulence, bloating, discomfort, and/or pain), or cause a more widespread toxicity in the body if they are absorbed. The result of either is poor availability of essential nutrients and an irritated gut, causing low energy and poor health.

HINTS FOR A HEALTHY DIGESTION

In addition to "food combining" there are several things you must do if you are to help your body digest and absorb your food properly.

1 Omit all refined foods, especially refined carbohydrates (white sugar, white flour, white pasta, etc.).

2 Omit all stimulants (including tea, coffee, colas, and chocolate).

3 Reduce sweet foods (honey, maple syrup, candy) to an absolute minimum.

4 Reduce alcohol to a minimum. Avoid drinking if possible.

5 Reduce total fat intake to a minimum and focus intake around seeds, nuts, virgin cold-pressed oils, and the oils in oily fish.

6 Reduce salt intake to a minimum, if necessary cutting out regular salt and changing to one of the "low salt" alternatives.

7 Eat good-quality live yogurt (containing beneficial bacteria) every day.

8 Chew your food thoroughly; take your time over eating; savor and enjoy each mouthful.

9 Don't eat when you are upset or stressed; wait until you are feeling calmer.

10 Don't drink fluids with your meals (this dilutes the digestive juices), or within a half hour either side of a meal. But make sure you still have a good intake of fluids each day.

LEFT *Slippery elm is a gentle and soothing digestive remedy.*

FOOD COMBINING

Many people with digestive problems try "food combining", known as the Hay Diet (after Dr Hay who first described this way of eating). The main principle is never to mix concentrated carbohydrates and concentrated proteins in the same meal, encouraging the digestion of one food group at a time.

When carbohydrates and proteins are broken down, they need different conditions for their enzymes to act correctly; the breakdown of carbohydrate requires a neutral environment, and that of protein takes place in an acid environment. By eating carbohydrates and proteins at different times you will promote ideal conditions for the complete breakdown of foods.

SUPPLEMENTS

There is a variety of supplements that assist in digestive healing; your nutritional therapist should be able to advise you, and may offer you a urine test to assess leaky gut levels. In general, you might like to try a supplement of digestive enzymes and hydrochloric acid capsules (avoid these supplements if you have ulcers or gastric disease).

Many supplements are available that encourage further healing of the digestive tract (such as slippery elm, cabagin, zinc, vitamin A), and others that will correct the bowel flora (*Lactobacillus acidophilus* and *Bifidobacterium* complex, burtyric acid, biotin and fructo-oligosaccharides. Quercetin, *Ginkgo biloba*, *Aloe vera* and antioxidant vitamins and minerals can reduce damage already caused to the gut.

Food Allergy and Intolerance

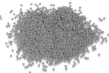

ABOVE *Gluten in grains, such as oats, can cause an allergic reaction.*

YOUR DIGESTION *may be fine (only one or two "yes" answers to the digestion questionnaire on the previous page), but you may still have some foods in your diet to which you are intolerant. Alternatively, you may have some digestive problems and be working on them, but at the same time need to assess your intolerance levels. Food intolerance can cause a general feeling of malaise, with an array of symptoms, ranging from migraines to skin irritations.*

Since even the best digestion is only about 50–60 percent efficient, this means that some undigested or partially digested food may be reaching the areas of absorption (mainly in the lower small intestine or ileum), and if the lining of this area is more porous than it should be (leaky gut), then fragments of partially digested protein can escape through to the blood where they are likely to be recognized as a "foreign invader" by the immune system. Those to whom this happens may then find they get the symptoms of an allergy or food intolerance.

In general, food allergy causes an adverse immune system reaction in which antibodies, or defensive proteins, are released to combat what the body perceives as an invasion by an enemy. A true allergic reaction can be measured by a blood test. It is usually immediate and triggered by a protein, e.g. gluten from grains or casein from milk.

Generally, we tend to call anything having an immediate reaction an "allergy", while anything having a delayed or masked reaction is an "intolerance", though the situation is complicated by the allergy to

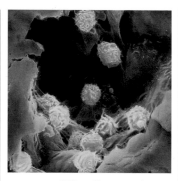

ABOVE *White cells may attack "foreign" protein in allergic reactions.*

gluten, celiac disease, which normally provokes a delayed response.

In this section we are mostly looking at intolerance since this is the more difficult to weed out. The more common foods causing intolerance are wheat, dairy foods, eggs, citrus fruit, chocolate, red wine, coffee, and nuts. The most likely will be those foods eaten regularly each day, which may cause an overall feeling of "just not quite right", with a few niggling little symptoms present most of the time.

Go through the checklist opposite to assess your level of intolerance. Score one point for each symptom, in any one of the groups, that you suffer from frequently.

ALLERGY QUESTIONNAIRE

Taking your score from the questionnaire opposite:
11 – 30 (with no more than three in one group) You seem to have a small amount of food intolerance. Try cutting out the main allergenic foods (wheat, dairy foods, eggs, citrus fruit, chocolate, red wine, coffee, and nuts) for two weeks and see if your "niggling" symptoms disappear. If they do, try adding each food back into your diet, one at a time. Eat your "test" food every day for three days, then leave a gap before you reintroduce the next food. Any food bringing a return of symptoms would be better avoided for a few months. **31 and over** (or four or more in any one group) You have a major problem with food intolerance. Consult a nutritionist about undertaking a hypoallergenic diet.

NOTE *There are no specific questions related to digestive symptoms since they have been assessed earlier.*

CHECKING FOR ALLERGIES AND FOOD INTOLERANCE

The following case study shows how you can work out if you have a reaction to a certain food or foods. You can apply the same questionnaire to yourself. Look at each group and score a point for each symptom that regularly applies to you. Then add up the totals. With less than 10 overall, and not more than two in any one group of six, you should have no worries. If you score more than 11, then follow the advice given in the box on the facing page.

Eyes and ears
Frequent itchy ears or earache/tinnitus/gritty, watery, or itchy eyes/swollen, sticky or red eyelids/permanent dark circles under the eyes/visual problems not related to definite eye defects.
TOM'S SCORE: **2**

Nose, mouth, and throat
Sinusitis, hay fever, or stuffy nose/sneezing attacks or excessive mucus production unrelated to a cold/irritating cough, not related to cigarette smoking or infection/constant sore or catarrhy throat, or hoarseness/halitosis (bad breath)/sore or cracked lips, mouth corners, tongue or receding gums.
TOM'S SCORE: **5**

Lungs and heart
Chestiness, wheeziness, or asthma/shortness of breath/high blood pressure/rapid heartbeat when resting/palpitations/general discomfort in chest area.
TOM'S SCORE: **2**

Head and emotions
Headaches and migraine/insomnia or restless sleep/behavioral changes or problems/mild depression/loss of humor/frequent irritability or aggressiveness/frequent anxiety or nervousness.
TOM'S SCORE: **1**

Mind
Frequent concentration and memory lapses/poor comprehension, or confusion/coordination problems, or learning difficulties/indecisiveness/stuttering, or inarticulation/obsessiveness or phobias.
TOM'S SCORE: **0**

Skin
Non-specific itchy skin/excessive sweating, or cold sweats/hot flashes, or "bloodshot" cheeks/non-specific rash, or dry skin/thinning hair or sudden hair loss/acne or psoriasis.
TOM'S SCORE: **3**

Energy, and activity levels
Apathy or sluggishness/unusual fatigue/lethargy/hyperactivity/inability to relax, restlessness/exhaustion after light exercise.
TOM'S SCORE: **3**

Joints and muscles
Generalized joint pain or stiffness/bursitis or arthritis/deep bone pain/weak or sore muscles/generalized muscle aches and pains/frequent muscle cramps.
TOM'S SCORE: **0**

Weight
Cravings (especially carbohydrates)/binge eating, compulsive eating, or comfort eating/alcohol cravings/fluid retention/weight fluctuation over a short period of time/excessive weight or underweight, resistant to change in diet.
TOM'S SCORE: **1**

TOM'S TOTAL SCORE: 17

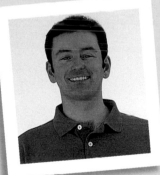

LEFT Tom scored 17 on the questionnaire. After eliminating dairy products from his diet he found that his symptoms disappeared.

NOTE *Many of the above symptoms can be associated with severe medical problems; always consult your own physician about anything that concerns you.*

Toxins

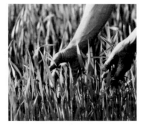

ABOVE *The environment is loaded with potential toxins, from air pollution to pesticides.*

FEW PEOPLE THINK *about the way the everyday chemicals they encounter may affect them. But toxins reach your liver and adipose (fatty connective) tissue through a variety of ways – in the water you drink, from the air both within your home and workplace, and from outside. We eat fruit and vegetables loaded with pesticide and chemical residues, and battery-farmed animals that are dosed up with antibiotics and artificial hormones. Moreover, dioxins, one of the most toxic groups of manmade substances ever made, are turning up in our milk, eggs, and fish.*

In addition to toxins that enter our bodies with our food, many physiological processes, particularly those reacting to stress, produce within the body metabolic by products that are toxic and could cause problems if not removed.

All of these many chemicals and metabolites in the blood supply and the tissues must be removed at a greater rate than the new ones are entering via our lungs and gut. Only then will we make headway in removing some of the toxic deposits that we may have had stored in our bodies for many years.

The body is constantly working to expel toxins through the liver, lungs, kidneys, skin, intestines, bowel, lymphatic, and immune systems in an attempt to achieve homeostasis (balance). The younger and healthier you are, the more effective this process is. But, as you get older or as your health deteriorates, this self-cleansing mechanism can become overloaded and you take in more toxins than you are able to remove.

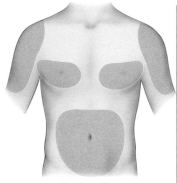

ABOVE *Toxins are often stored in fatty tissues under the skin, or in the joints.*

The body ensures that poisonous substances it is unable to detoxify and remove from the tissues are locked away, at least initially, where they can do least damage to the system. This usually means surrounding them in fat and storing them away in the adipose tissue under the skin, or in fatty tissues surrounding major organs like the heart and kidneys. Some people seem to store their toxins in joints, and consequently suffer from joint and muscle pain, and stiffness.

A toxic system is also an acidic one and to function effectively the body needs a neutral to slightly alkaline environment. Lightening the toxic load with a full detoxification program will cause your body to become more alkaline.

Alternatively, you could take detoxification more slowly by carrying on with the New Pyramid program and having just one full day a week on a cleansing regime. Or you could do a type of "split" cleanse by having fresh fruit only (organic, if possible) for breakfast every morning and only filtered or bottled water, or herb tea. More fruit can be eaten throughout the morning if desired, and then from lunchtime onward, you can return to your main diet.

This "split" program is designed to fit in with your daily detoxification cycle, where for around eight hours from, say 4:00 a.m. until 12:00 noon, the body is cleansing itself naturally. Then from around 12 noon, the next eight hours is the "intake" period when you will be eating your normal healthy diet. The last eight-hour period from around 8:00 p.m. is the "assimilation" period when your body is digesting and delivering nutrients.

Many good combinations of herbs and nutrients will expedite toxin removal, and damp down some of the more unpleasant healing reactions that may occur. Ask any good health store for advice about these detoxification formulas, or consult a nutritional therapist.

WARNING

There are some individuals who should not detoxify. If you have an eating disorder, a serious mental problem, are pregnant or breastfeeding, are currently taking prescription medication, or are at all concerned about any preexisting condition, do not attempt a detoxification diet without taking the advice of your medical practitioner.

TOXINS CAN GATHER IN
THE KNEE JOINT

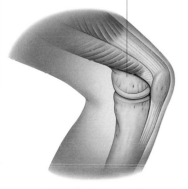

ABOVE *Toxins are sometimes deposited in the joints, creating pain and stiffness.*

WORKING OUT
YOUR TOXIN LEVEL

Simple "yes" and "no" answers are required to the following questions. They assume you have done some healing work on your digestion and intestines and have worked on any food intolerances you may have had.

❀ Do you feel sluggish or dull-headed much of the time and find concentrating difficult?

❀ Is your energy level low in the morning and again about 3:00 p.m.?

❀ Do you have bad breath, or an unpleasant taste in your mouth most of the time?

❀ Do you have strong body/foot odor?

❀ Do you seem to need excessive amounts of sleep (more than eight hours per night)?

❀ Do you have a poor tolerance to alcohol?

❀ Do you feel the cold more than others?

❀ Do you often have discomfort in the right upper abdomen (around lower ribs) or under the right shoulder blade?

❀ Do you have bowel movements less than once daily?

❀ Are your stools yellow, clay-colored, or foul-smelling?

❀ Do you suffer from chronic constipation?

❀ Do you have joint pains?

❀ Is your skin dull/dry/greasy/spotty?

❀ Do you consume more than two units of alcohol per day?

❀ Do you develop indigestion and/or headaches in response to eating fat-based foods?

❀ Do onions, cucumbers, radishes, or cabbage cause digestive distress?

❀ Do you have a poor appetite?

❀ Do you feel nauseous frequently?

❀ Do you get itchy skin with no apparent cause?

❀ Do you have asthma, eczema, hay fever, or other allergic conditions?

SCORING

Score one point for each "yes" answer

3 and over You will need to cleanse (detoxify) your system before returning to a basic wholesome diet such as the New Pyramid program. The more questions you have answered in the affirmative, the greater your need to detoxify. Consult a nutritional therapist about undertaking a detoxification diet. A three-day stint would suffice in a mild case or the time can be extended by two-day sessions if needed, through to a minimum of 11 days or, only in extreme cases, 13 days.

DETOXIFICATION AND THE LIVER

The organ that is primarily responsible for removing toxic products as they flow through the blood is the liver. Detoxification in the liver is controlled by two phases.

Phase one of detoxification (oxidation) involves the activity of a special family of enzymes known as the P450s, whose job it is to activate a fat-soluble toxin and make it more able to be dissolved in bodily fluids. The nutrients needed to support a healthy oxidation phase are vitamins B_2, B_3, B_6, B_{12}, folic acid, vitamin C, bioflavonoids (such as rutin from buckwheat, hesperidin from citrus, and quercetin from onions and garlic), vitamin E, glutathione, branched-chain amino acids, and phospholipids, plus a good supply of antioxidant nutrients to disarm free radicals created during this phase. Some people have problems if this first phase works too well, and a lot of free radicals are produced, which are highly toxic to the body. Such people are called "pathological detoxifiers" and they can get worse when put on

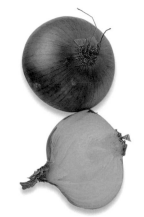

ABOVE *Onion is a source of the bioflavonoids that are necessary for proper oxidation, which is the first phase of detoxification.*

a supplement program, especially if polyunsaturated oils are given; so take care (detoxification phases one and two can be assessed by stool and/or urine samples taken by your nutritional therapist).

Phase two of detoxification (conjugation) is where the toxin is combined with another molecule, making it less destructive. This phase can also be stimulated back into activity by certain nutrients, such as the B-complex vitamins (especially B_5), beta-carotene, vitamins C and E, molybdenum, selenium, manganese, copper, zinc, glutathione, and the amino acids L-cysteine, L-methionine, L-acetyl cysteine, L-glycine, L-glutamine, and taurine, plus a diet that decreases the toxic load. There are many herbs that are good at nourishing the liver tissue and increasing the activity of both phases of detoxification – two excellent examples are dandelion, and milk thistle.

The kidneys are also involved in detoxification since they filter the blood and remove toxic wastes that

have not been released by the liver into the bile. There are several botanicals, such as celery seeds, alfalfa, parsley, etc. that will help strengthen the kidneys.

A qualified nutritional therapist should be able to arrange for a test to assess your phase one and phase two detoxification capacity. This non-invasive test uses dietary "challenges", testing their breakdown products in the urine.

One further important point to mention is that the liver is unable to remove toxins stored in other body tissues and organs, since it can only remove toxins from the blood as it passes through. We need, therefore, something to remove any stored poisonous substances retained by cells and not released into the blood. This is sometimes referred to as "stage one" in the detoxification process (this is different from phase one in the liver), and a diet high in fresh organically grown vegetables and fruit, and filtered water, would usually achieve this. Once the toxins are out of the cells and flowing around the body in the blood, the liver (always assuming it has the energy and capacity to do this) is

BELOW *Milk thistle is one of several herbs that regenerate liver tissue.*

WARNING

Do not move onto a detoxification program until you have done some work on improving your digestion, healing your gut lining, rebalancing your gut flora, and removing a large proportion of your food intolerances; otherwise, toxins released in cleansing may further irritate the absorptive lining, or may be reabsorbed.

then able to remove them by detoxification into the bile, which then enters the alimentary canal at the duodenum. From here, the toxins can travel the length of the intestines and pass out of the body. This is "stage two" of detoxification, it is helped by foods such as wholegrain brown rice.

It is, unfortunately, while we have toxins circulating around in our blood that we get symptoms of detoxification, sometimes referred to as a "healing reaction". The list of possible detoxification symptoms is long but usually includes things like a fuzzy head, coated tongue, sweating, fever, increased bowel movements and urination, rash, reduced energy, and weight loss. If any of these sound familiar, it is because they are similar to the symptoms of food intolerance. But intolerance is also a reaction that stimulates the body in trying to rid itself of these "allergens". How do

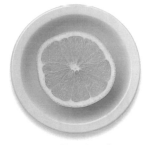

ABOVE *Parsley nourishes the kidneys and aids detoxification.*

you tell the difference between the two? Are you intolerant to a food or foods in your diet, or are you toxic and going through a healing crisis? The only thing that will give you the right answer is to take a careful look at your diet. If you had food intolerances and you have mostly cleared them through a hypoallergenic diet, or an elimination diet given to you by your therapist, and you are actively engaged upon a detoxification diet, then your symptoms will be those of

ABOVE *Grapefruit alone is not enough for detoxification*

detoxification. If you have, as yet, made no attempt to remove any food intolerances you have, and are on a detoxification diet, then your symptoms will also be those of detoxification, since detoxification diets in general are extremely low in allergens. If you have, as yet, made no attempt to do either of these things (that is, remove intolerances or detoxify), then you may be suffering from symptoms of food intolerance and a high toxic load. Your body is just reacting to the substances circulating around in your blood.

A detoxification diet that is poorly balanced, for example, one that involves eating a grapefruit at every meal for several days, will not give good results. Since there is no fibrous food passing through the intestines to enable efficient toxin removal from the body, a large proportion of the stage one toxins are simply reabsorbed. The sufferer in this case probably goes through some unpleasant detoxification symptoms without benefitting.

RIGHT *The liver and kidneys work together in making fuel available to the body, as well as being prime centers for detoxification.*

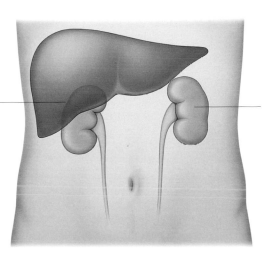

THE LIVER PROCESSES NUTRIENTS FROM THE INTESTINES, AS WELL AS REMOVING TOXINS FROM THE BLOOD

THE KIDNEYS FILTER OUT THE WASTES IN THE BLOOD PRODUCED BY THE LIVER'S WORK

Pollution

IN ADDITION TO removing toxins that may have been stored in your body for a long time, you may also like to consider the general level of pollution in your home or workplace. There is not a lot of point in going through a thorough cleansing program, only to replace body toxins with environmental ones.

Living or working in an area where there are a large number of airborne chemicals will put your detoxification system under stress and will use up important energy that you could put to better use. Of course, there will always be a limit; there is very little we can do about general air pollution in the street, and even in our workplace there may be very little we can do to make the air we breathe less chemically laden. Thankfully, many offices, work areas and public places are now designated nonsmoking areas, and new governmental regulations, such as the C.O.S.H.H. (Control of Substances Hazardous to Health) in Britain, and government protection agencies, such as the Environmental Protection Agency (E.P.A.) in the U.S., puts the responsibility onto the employer to control any chemically damaging substances.

On an individual level, you can assess the number of airborne pollutants, such as insecticides, aerosol sprays, varnishes, and air fresheners, in your own home, by answering the questionnaire opposite.

TOP The Whitaker family's house was revealed to have a very high level of chemical contamination when they filled out the questionnaire.

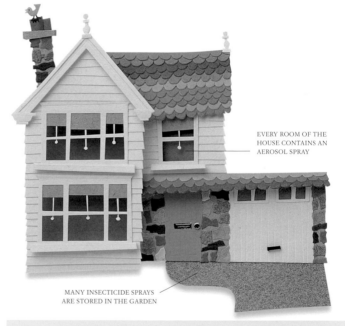

EVERY ROOM OF THE HOUSE CONTAINS AN AEROSOL SPRAY

MANY INSECTICIDE SPRAYS ARE STORED IN THE GARDEN

POLLUTANTS QUESTIONNAIRES

Taking your score from the questionnaires opposite:

0 – 50 The chemical contamination of your home is low, and well below average.

51 – 100 You are a moderate user of chemicals, but you err on the side of having too many. Make sure you dispose, safely, of those you really don't need. Focus particularly on any products that make any members of your family sneeze or feel unwell.

101 – 150 The level of chemical contamination of your home is high and is likely to cause you problems. Safely dispose of those items you know you can really do without, and restrict the use of those that you feel are vital.

151 and over Your home is heavily contaminated with chemicals. Take stock of all those items you really do need, and safely dispose of the rest.

CHECKING FOR POLLUTANTS

When the Whitaker family completed this questionnaire, they were shocked by the level of pollutants in their home. See how you compare to the Whitakers – score as indicated at the end of each question.

QUESTIONNAIRE 1

1 Count all the aerosol sprays in your home, garage and/or garden shed (include any polishes and other cleaning materials, hair sprays, air fresheners, deodorants, shaving creams, starch laundry sprays.
Total number of aerosols: 10
SCORE 1 POINT EACH:
WHITAKER FAMILY: **10**

2 Count any insecticidal pet shampoos and flea collars used in the last three months, and any pesticides or insecticides used in the garden in the last three months.
Total number of insecticides: 2
SCORE 2 POINTS EACH:
WHITAKER FAMILY: **4**

3 Count all the times you have brought "dry-cleaned" clothes into the house, or have had any furnishings (carpets, curtains, upholstery) dry-cleaned, or used dry-cleaning treatments in the house or car, in the last six months.
Total number of dry-cleaned items: 5
SCORE 2 POINTS EACH:
WHITAKER FAMILY: **10**

4 Count the number of long-lasting air fresheners or deodorizers in the kitchen, bathroom, or car.
Total number of long-lasting air fresheners: 2
SCORE 2 POINTS EACH:
WHITAKER FAMILY: **4**

5 Count the number of gas fires, gas heaters, gas cooker, paraffin heaters, or bottled gas heaters you have in your house and garage.
Total number of gas appliances: 2
SCORE 2 POINTS EACH:
WHITAKER FAMILY: **4**

6 Count the number of flexible plastic items, such as shower curtains, tablecloths, etc.
Total number of flexible plastic items: 7
SCORE 4 POINTS EACH:
WHITAKER FAMILY: **28**

7 Count the number of occasions on which you have carried out any decorating in the house (especially if you did the work yourself) within the last three months.
Total number of decorating occasions: 0
SCORE 5 POINTS EACH:
WHITAKER FAMILY: **0**

8 Count how many long-lasting insecticides are used in the house, garage, or car.
Total number of long-lasting insecticides: 3
SCORE 5 POINTS EACH:
WHITAKER FAMILY: **15**

9 Count the number of times you have used cellulose paints or paint/varnish strippers in the house or garage within the last two months.
Total number of times strippers used: 0
SCORE 5 POINTS EACH:
WHITAKER FAMILY: **0**

10 Count the number of items of plastic-covered furniture in your house or garage.
Total number of furniture: 2
SCORE 5 POINTS EACH:
WHITAKER FAMILY: **10**

TOTAL SO FAR: 85 POINTS

QUESTIONNAIRE 2

Add on the following scores, if applicable:
● Do you have a new car?
SCORE 4 POINTS
WHITAKER FAMILY: **0**
● Do you use strong-smelling glues in the house?
SCORE 4 POINTS
WHITAKER FAMILY: **4**
● Do you use biological laundry detergents (those that contain enzymes), regularly?
SCORE 5 POINTS:
WHITAKER FAMILY: **5**
● Do you use fabric softeners in your washing regularly?
SCORE 5 POINTS
WHITAKER FAMILY: **5**
● Do you have urea-formaldehyde cavity foam insulation in your home or garage?
SCORE 10 POINTS
WHITAKER FAMILY: **10**
● Can you smell gas anywhere in the house?
SCORE 20 POINTS
WHITAKER FAMILY: **0**
● Have you had the woodwork in your home treated with preservative within the past year?
SCORE 25 POINTS
WHITAKER FAMILY: **0**

SUBTOTAL: 24 POINTS
(additional points)

GRAND TOTAL: 109 POINTS
(pollution points)

Blood-sugar Balance

THE LEVEL OF *"sugar" (glucose) in the blood is under the control of a pair of hormones called insulin and glucagon. Both are manufactured in the pancreas. When the amounts of the two hormones are unbalanced, the person begins to suffer from fatigue.*

The pancreas secretes insulin into the bloodstream after a meal containing carbohydrate. The insulin travels to the liver and the muscles, instructing them to take excess glucose from the bloodstream and to store it as glycogen. As insulin levels increase, blood-glucose levels start to fall, but when this reaches a critical low level, it causes the brain to send for more supplies. If these instructions from the brain are ignored or slow in being fulfilled, you begin to suffer symptoms of "hypoglycemia", the first of which is usually mental fatigue.

Under normal circumstances (where some carbohydrate is properly balanced with protein), when a small drop in glucose occurs, the hormone glucagon is released from the pancreas and stimulates the breakdown of glycogen stores in the liver to release glucose into the blood again. A possible problem arises here if you are using a food combining diet where you do not eat carbohydrate and protein at the same meal. In this case, you must insure that each day you have one protein meal (preferably at lunchtime), and one carbohydrate meal (preferably at supper time), and one neutral meal of low G.I. (glycemic index, see opposite) fruit and seeds. Blood-sugar will then be balanced out well over the day.

In addition to the insulin–glucagon seesaw, the release of the hormone adrenaline from the adrenal glands, and the release of the glucocorticoids (from the adrenal cortex) occurs as a response to stress. These hormones also raise blood-sugar levels by further stimulation of the pancreas and liver.

Continued high stress levels from mental, emotional, or nutritional sources do not require a physical response ("fight" or "flight"). The energy that has been made available to combat stress is returned to storage as glycogen or fat.

If blood-sugar levels stay low, a part of the brain called the hypothalamus is stimulated and we feel hungry, encouraging us to replenish our sugar level in the blood. Constant consumption of poorly balanced meals (too much carbohydrate in relation to protein) destroys the fine balance in the blood-sugar homeostasis.

If we regularly consume sweet foods and carbohydrates with a high G.I., this will cause a surge of insulin into the blood to deal with the excess sugar. The pancreas may react to the large amounts of glucose entering the system by producing too much insulin, causing blood-sugar levels to drop. We begin to feel hungry and tired, reach for something sweet, and the vicious cycle continues.

LEFT *When we are stressed but not able to respond with "fight or flight", the extra glucose is converted to fat.*

GLYCEMIC INDEX OF SOME COMMON CARBOHYDRATE-RICH FOODS

HIGH GLYCEMIC INDEX	(OVER 70)	MODERATE GLYCEMIC INDEX	(50 – 70)	LOW GLYCEMIC INDEX	(UNDER 50)
Glucose	100	Pancakes	70	Porridge (oatmeal)	49
Maltose	100	White bread	70	Natural wheatbran	
Cooked parsnips	97	Fresh mashed potato	70	breakfast cereal	49
Sports drinks		Watermelon	70	Chocolate	48
(glucose drinks)	95	Wholewheat bread	69	Baked beans (no sugar)	48
Cooked carrots	92	Rye crispbread	69	Dried peas	47
Boiled white rice	88	Croissant	68	Yam (sweet potato)	42
Honey	87	Soft drinks	68	Wholewheat spaghetti	41
Baked potato	85	Shredded breakfast		Boiled white pasta	41
Cornflakes	84	cereal (wheat)	67	Apple juice	40
Instant mashed potato	83	Granola or muesli		Oranges	37
Wheat breakfast cereal	75	(unsweetened)	66	Wholewheat pasta	
Bagel	72	Brown rice	66	(boiled)	36
Millet	71	Cordial/fruit		Butterbeans	36
		concentrate	66	Garbanzo beans	36
		Sucrose (sugar)	64	Apples, pears	35
		Raisins	64	Ice cream (full-fat)	34
		Cooked beets	62	Flavored yogurt	34
		Boiled new potatoes	61	Whole milk	33
		Ice cream (low-fat)	60	Black-eyed peas	32
		Banana	59	Skim milk	31
		Pastry	59	Haricot beans	30
		Crackers or digestives	59	Lentils	29
		Potato chips (full-fat)	59	Kidney beans	20
		Corn (sweetcorn)	58	Fructose (fruit sugar)	20
		Basmati rice (brown)	56	Soybeans	15
		Whole boiled potato			
		(with skin)	56		
		Sultanas	55		
		Rich tea cookies	54		
		Oatmeal cookies	52		
		Orange juice	51		
		Garden peas	51		
		Buckwheat	50		
		Rye bread	50		
		White spaghetti	50		

CORNFLAKES

HONEY

WHITE RICE

SPORTS DRINK

YAMS (SWEET POTATOES)

BLACK-EYED PEAS

Blood-sugar Control

SEVERAL FOODS THAT *many modern diets are based on, such as potatoes, white rice, and other grains, cooked carrots, fruit juice, and low-sugar breakfast cereals, have a high G.I., and may be causing problems with blood-sugar control. If suboptimum blood-sugar control is a problem, you might consider taking supplements in addition to changing to low G.I. foods.*

HELPFUL SUPPLEMENTS

As with all other aspects of our physiology, certain nutritional supplements can help to nourish specific parts of the body, allowing it to recover more quickly than it does by diet alone. In the case of suboptimum blood-sugar control, the main nutrients are the B-complex vitamins, since it is these substances that help to metabolize carbohydrates effectively within the body. Although it consists of individual vitamins that are distinguished from each other by number, the whole B-vitamin complex works in unison, which is why the vitamins are grouped together rather than put into separate classes. It is therefore unlikely to be of benefit, and may cause a greater imbalance, if any of the B vitamins are taken separately from the rest of the complex. If you feel you need one specific B vitamin more than the others, take a B-complex vitamin, plus at the same time, extra of any one particular B vitamin that you feel you need.

In addition, G.T.F. (glucose tolerance factor) can be supplemented either in the form of additional G.T.F. or as a more general dietary supplement containing chromium. Other helpful supplements include the antioxidants (vitamins A, C, E), the minerals manganese and zinc, high potency garlic, lecithin, E.P.A. (eicosapentaenoic acid from fish), and spirulina. If in doubt, ask a nutritional therapist or health food store for advice. See your physician first if you are diabetic.

BLOOD-SUGAR CONTROL

If you have health problems that originate in poor blood-sugar control, you need to cut out from your diet all foods with a high glycemic content, and for a while also avoid those with a moderate glycemic content. After about a month or so you can reintroduce the moderate ones, but only one at a time, and giving each one three days before adding another one (to assess suitability).

DAY ONE	DAY FOUR	DAY SEVEN
Rye crispbread has a glycemic index of 69	Orange juice has a glycemic index of 51	Corn has a glycemic index of 58

BLOOD-SUGAR QUESTIONNAIRE

To check how stable your blood sugar is, answer "yes" or "no" to the following questions.

❁ Do you get tired and/or hungry in the mid-afternoon?

❁ About an hour or two after eating a full meal that includes dessert, do you find yourself wanting more of the dessert?

❁ Is it harder for you to control your eating for the rest of the day if you have breakfast containing carbohydrates than it is if you have only coffee or a meal rich in protein instead?

❁ When you want to lose weight, do you find it easier not to eat for most of the day than to try to eat several small diet meals?

❁ Once you start eating candy, starches, or snack foods, do you often find difficulty stopping?

❁ If you are feeling low, does a snack of cake or cookies make you feel better?

❁ If there are potatoes, bread, pasta, or dessert on the table, do you often skip eating vegetables or salad?

❁ Do you frequently get severe mood swings for no apparent reason?

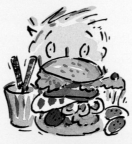

BEDTIME SNACKING

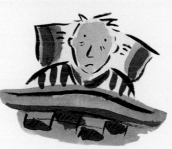

NIGHTTIME HUNGER

ABOVE *Waking in the night and needing food is a symptom of bloodsugar irregularities*

❁ Do you feel sleepy (with a feeling as if you were "drugged") after eating a large meal containing bread/pasta/potatoes or dessert, but on the other hand feel more energetic after a meal that consists only of protein and salad?

❁ Do you often wake in the middle of the night feeling hungry and are unable to get back to sleep without eating something?

❁ If you are going to eat at a friend's house, do you sometimes eat a small snack before you go in case dinner is delayed?

❁ At a restaurant, do you find yourself eating too much bread before the meal is served?

❁ Do you get attacks of sweating for no reason?

❁ When you haven't eaten for a few hours, do you ever get dizzy or shaky?

❁ Do you ever feel as if you are going to pass out or are unable to think clearly if you have gone without food for a few hours?

❁ When hungry do you mainly crave sugary things?

SCORING

Score one point for each "yes" answer.

0 – 3 Your blood-sugar control appears to be working fairly well, and you could safely include complex carbohydrates of a high G.I. in your New Pyramid Food program.

4 – 10 It is likely that at least some of the time you have a problem maintaining the correct sugar balance, and you would do well to steer clear of sweet foods and those carbohydrates with a high G.I. for a period of around one to two months. Concentrate your carbohydrates around brown rice, buckwheat, lentils, beans, oats, wholewheat spaghetti, and low G.I. fruit and vegetables.

11 and over Poor blood-sugar control is certainly one of the things causing your ill health. Remove all refined and processed foods from your diet. Also avoid carbohydrate foods with a high G.I., and restrict very severely those with a moderate G.I. for a month or two.

Stress

IF YOU FEEL *that stress from emotional problems, relationships, or your work environment is sabotaging your nutritional healing attempts, by causing excessive (or comfort) eating, or causing you to indulge too frequently in alcohol, try the quick test below to assess to what degree you may be affected.*

HOW STRESSED ARE YOU?

Answer "yes" or "no" to the following questions.

- Is your energy level lower than it used to be?
- Are you especially competitive at work, sports, or relationships?
- Do you feel you work harder than most of your colleagues?
- Do you find yourself often doing several tasks at the same time?
- Do you get very impatient if people or circumstances delay you?
- Do you feel guilty each time you try to relax?

- Do you become angry easily?
- Do you have a constant need to achieve, and for people to recognize your achievements?
- Do you have difficulty getting off to sleep, or do you sleep poorly/lightly, do you wake up with your mind racing?
- Do you often bottle up your thoughts and feelings?
- Are you always in a hurry to get somewhere, or get something done?

- Are there any long-term stressful situations in your life (parents, marriage, job, children, finances, etc.)?
- Has anyone very close to you died recently?
- Have you recently been divorced or separated from your partner?
- Have you had to leave a job recently?
- Have you moved house recently?
- Do you have poor self-image, low self-esteem, or low self-confidence?

SCORING

Score one point for each "yes" answer.

0 – 4 Stress effects on your health are low.

5 – 10 Your moderate stress levels are probably contributing to your health problems. Continue with a good wholefood diet such as the New Pyramid program, and insure that you consume maximum levels of antioxidant fruit and vegetables. Also, make sure you are taking a high-potency antioxidant supplement. Read on and carry out the Adrenal Function questionnaire on page 63, to assess just how much effect stress is having on your hormonal system.

11 and over It is almost certain that your stressful existence is a major cause of your health problems. Continue with this section and undertake the Adrenal Function questionnaire.

LEFT *Stress often makes us eat badly, but a good diet can help us cope with stress.*

LEFT *Stress can arise from any situation in our lives, and when we feel under stress it generally permeates all our activities, even those that are meant to help us unwind.*

PRESSURE OF WORK IS A PRIME CAUSE OF STRESS

EMOTIONAL PROBLEMS CAN COLOR OUR EVERY MOMENT

WHEN TENSE WE OFTEN FEEL WE HAVE NO CONTROL

STRESS PRODUCES A FEELING OF BEING CRUSHED

STRESS AND THE ENDOCRINE SYSTEM

Our ability to deal with stress is under the control of the endocrine (hormonal) system. Stress induces a series of reactions known as the "fight or flight" mechanism. Body systems act in a coordinated fashion in order to prepare the body for sudden physical action and energy expenditure.

The first, immediate effect is caused by the brain stimulating a part of the adrenal glands called the adrenal medulla to secrete the hormone adrenaline. This hormone acts on the liver, stimulating it to convert some of its stored glycogen to glucose, and causing it to release this into the bloodstream. Blood pressure and heart rate increase to allow this "emergency" glucose to be conveyed around the system to the target cells. The breathing rate is similarly increased in order to bring in the necessary extra oxygen to deal with the breakdown of glucose for energy release. Digestion stops as the blood supply is diverted to the muscles to prepare them to move quickly away from the "source of danger". The blood platelets get ready to aggregate quickly in case they need to form a blood clot over any cut or wound.

In addition to this, stress stimulates the pituitary gland to release a hormone called A.C.T.H. (adrenocorticotrophic hormone), and this hormone stimulates the adrenal cortex to release a group of hormones called the glucocorticoids and mineralocorticoids. The glucocorticoids further help in making glucose available to the cells, while the mineralocorticoids help to retain sodium, which is needed by the body for increased nervous transmission and for appropriate muscle contraction.

LEFT AND BELOW *Time can tyrannize us, causing active stress, while money worries are a very common cause of stress.*

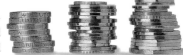

HORMONE EXHAUSTION AND STRESS REDUCTION

The "fight or flight" mechanism was necessary to enable the body to deal quickly with dangerous situations. In modern humans, although the physiological reaction to stress remains the same, the triggers and the effect are completely different. The cumulative physiological reactions to raise blood glucose, blood pressure, heart rate, breathing rate, and blood-clotting mechanisms, which are precursors to rapid physical activity, still occur, but we rarely choose to fight or run away. Since the majority of our stress triggers are an impossible workload, worries about money, frustrations in slow-moving traffic, demanding children, and unsympathetic partners, we rarely do anything "physical" with the extra energy we have at our disposal, except perhaps fume, swear, and shout. The cumulative effect of stress hormones, stress triggers, and a heightened response level can eventually lead to anxiety states or will simply keep the body on "red alert".

All of these factors can eventually lead to exhaustion of several endocrine (hormonal) glands and in particular the adrenals. There is a slowing down of the metabolic rate as the adrenals and other endocrine glands, such as the pancreas and the thyroid, begin to function less well. This inevitably leads to a general slowing-down of the whole system, the accumulation of weight, and a worsening ability to fight off disease and cancers.

Nevertheless, a little stress is good for us. It keeps us sharp and on our toes, and it does stimulate metabolism in the short term.

HORMONAL BALANCE

The nutritional aspects of stress reduction are based on the maintenance of hormonal output. Adrenal hormones, such as adrenaline and cortisol, are the prime contenders in stress reactions, as too are insulin from the pancreas and thyroxine from the thyroid. Another hormone called D.H.E.A. (dehydroepiandrosterone), manufactured in the body from cholesterol, is intimately involved in glucose metabolism and the stress response, and has been heralded as "the youth hormone". When homeostatic equilibrium involving all the hormones related to stress handling is absent, there is a gradual progression through states of chronic stress adaptation to the exhaustion of many glands.

Hormonal balance is of vital importance in preventing stressful events resulting in glandular exhaustion, and is best achieved by eating a well-balanced, wholefood diet. The omission of refined and processed foods, together with stimulants such as tea, coffee, salt, and sugar, is important when optimizing nutrition to combat stress. Stimulant foods artificially raise pancreatic activity leading to a chaotic chemical state.

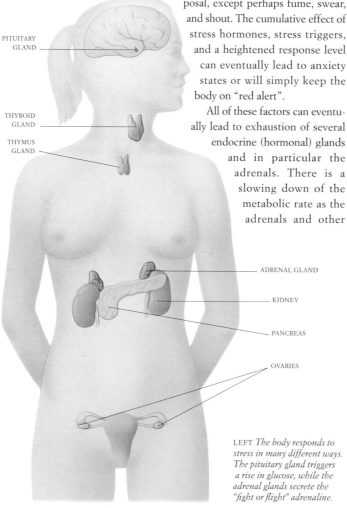

PITUITARY GLAND

THYROID GLAND

THYMUS GLAND

ADRENAL GLAND

KIDNEY

PANCREAS

OVARIES

LEFT *The body responds to stress in many different ways. The pituitary gland triggers a rise in glucose, while the adrenal glands secrete the "fight or flight" adrenaline.*

ADRENAL STRESS QUESTIONNAIRE

*If you feel that stress has been a big feature in your life for a long period of time, give "yes" or "no"
answers to the following questions, which are based on symptoms of suboptimum adrenal function.*

- Do you have a tendency to severe emotional swings?
- Do you have a tendency toward allergy-related conditions, e.g. eczema, urticaria (hives), or hay fever?
- Do you have low blood pressure, or do you feel dizzy when standing up quickly?

- Do you feel unable to get enough air, i.e. feel suffocated, and frequently sigh or yawn?
- Do you feel lacking in energy in the morning and perhaps require a stimulant such as coffee or a cigarette to "get you going"?
- Are you sensitive to bright lights?

- Do you frequently have a dry mouth, lacking in saliva?
- Do your ankles swell, especially at night?
- Do you crave salty foods, such as chips, salty meats, salted nuts, etc.?
- Does eating foods such as cabbage, beans, or very starchy/sugary foods, give you indigestion?

SCORING

Score one point for each "yes" answer.

4 and over It is very likely that your protracted stress levels have reduced the efficiency of your adrenal glands to some degree. Supplementing your diet with nutrients such as vitamin C, the B-complex vitamins, and additional vitamin B$_5$ (usually in the form of calcium pantothenate), together with special adrenal nourishing herbs like Siberian ginseng, would be of real help. If you are considering consulting a nutritional therapist, he/she will be able to take non-invasive saliva samples for analysis of your adrenal stress index.

The best diet for anyone with high stress levels is the New Pyramid program, since this will not only nourish the endocrine system in general, but the feel-good factor inherent in this diet will itself promote better stress-handling. Metabolism-enhancing exercise will deal with increased levels of stress hormones as enhanced levels of endorphins, the pleasure molecules, are released.

Remember too, that high body toxicity and/or working and living in areas of high pollution will add chemical stress factors to the overall stress load. You would be well advised to combat toxicity and pollution problems first, by undergoing a detoxification program and depolluting your house. This will automatically give you more energy to deal with your emotional stress producers.

RIGHT *Regular exercise
puts the body in a condition
where moderate stress can
actually make you feel good.*

Thyroid Function

THE RATE OF METABOLISM *is controlled by the thyroid gland, which is positioned at the base of the throat. The thyroid gland produces and secretes the hormone thyroxine, in response to another hormone called T.S.H., which is made in the anterior pituitary gland. The pituitary gland controls metabolism and will be encouraged to raise metabolism by a stress reaction, exercise, or taking a stimulant food/beverage such as chocolate or coffee. However, despite the apparent usefulness of an increase in metabolic rate by these three means, a continually stimulated pituitary will eventually begin to underfunction.*

ABOVE *Wheat intolerance can impair thyroid function.*

As well as raising the metabolic level, the pituitary gland depresses metabolism when the person is on a calorie-reduced diet, or is fasting. This enables the body to conserve its stores of body fat. In these conditions the pituitary reduces the amount of T.S.H. that it sends to the thyroid gland, which has the effect of lessening thyroid output.

In normal circumstances, a finely tuned system will allow proper maintenance of metabolic rate appropriate to requirements at a particular time. However, there is much information available now which indicates that around 40 percent or more of the present population are suffering from some degree of thyroid malfunction. Research undertaken on thyroid conditions has indicated that many of them are likely to be due to food intolerance. Common food intolerances (particularly to the proteins in cow's milk and wheat) may be linked to the negative effect that allergens have on the thyroid gland, preventing it from working properly

and in consequence lowering the metabolic rate.

An underactive thyroid is generally characterized by weight increase (despite a reduction in appetite), slow pulse rate, sluggish digestion, constipation, lethargy, and apathy, and an over-susceptibility to the cold. An overactive thyroid usually occurs because of proliferation of thyroxine-producing cells within the thyroid, and results in

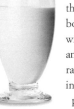

ABOVE *It is now thought that an intolerance to cow's milk can stop the thyroid working properly.*

the speeding up of the metabolic rate. This usually brings with it a drop in weight and an increase in appetite, more rapid digestion and diarrhea, increased heart and blood pressure, muscular tremors, nervous excitability, and apprehension.

Complete the questionnaires on pages 65 and 66 to establish how your thyroid is working and refer to the dietary recommendations overleaf.

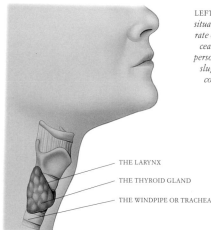

LEFT *The thyroid gland, which is situated in the throat, governs the rate of metabolism. If the thyroid ceases to function altogether, a person will become very tired and sluggish, and if not treated the condition will become fatal.*

THE LARYNX

THE THYROID GLAND

THE WINDPIPE OR TRACHEA

DO YOU SUFFER FROM AN UNDERACTIVE THYROID?

You can obtain some idea of your thyroid function by answering the following questions. Again, a simple "yes" or "no" is required, then consult the scoring box underneath.

- Do you tend to gain weight easily and fail to lose it even with a calorie-restricted diet?
- Are you chronically or frequently constipated?
- Is your skin pale, thick, dry, wrinkled, "waxy", or puffy, especially around the eyes?
- Do you feel lethargic, dull, confused, or uninterested much of the time?
- Is the hair on the outer third of your eyebrows noticeably thin or even absent?

- Is your hair thinning or falling out?
- Do you tend to feel better in the mornings and worse in the afternoons?
- Are you very sensitive to cold, or have cold hands and/or feet?
- Do you have ringing in the ears, or have you noticed any hearing loss?
- Is your appetite very poor, yet you are not losing weight?
- Is your pulse rate slow (below 65 beats per minute)?
- Do you have weakness and aches in your muscles?

- Do you often feel depressed?
- Do you have problems with menstruation or fertility?
- Have you lost interest in sex?
- Do you have headaches with focusing problems?
- Do you have sticky eyelids, slow healing, or frequent infections (especially of the throat)?
- Do you have tingling in your hands and feet?
- Have you noticed any changes in skin pigmentation?
- Do you have very brittle nails?

SCORING

Score one point for each "yes" answer.

If you have said "yes" to more than half of these questions, you may be suffering from an underactive thyroid (hypothyroidism). One self-test you might try before taking the matter further is to carry out the basal temperature test (see below). If you are concerned about a large proportion of the above symptoms, and your basal body temperature is low, see your physician, who will give you a thorough examination and may carry out a blood test to assess the level of your thyroid activity.

TEMPERATURE TEST

This test must be performed before you get out of bed and before you have undertaken any form of activity. It must be done before you drink or eat anything.

1 Place a thermometer under your right arm, insuring the "bulb" of the thermometer is exactly in the center of the underarm.
2 Keep the thermometer in place according to instructions.
3 Record the temperature as accurately as you can, to the smallest fraction of a degree.
4 Repeat this daily. If you are a regularly menstruating female, then the best time to do this is from day one of the menstrual cycle, for about a week. If you are a non-menstruating female or are male, you need to take your temperature over a period of two weeks.
5 Add up all your temperatures over the period and divide by the number of readings to obtain your average (mean) basal temperature.

The normal body temperature value is 98.6° to 99°F (36.8° to 37°C), so the more you depart from this value, the more likely there is to be a thyroid imbalance.
Underactive (hypothyroid) shows up as below the normal level, and overactive (hyperthyroid) as above the normal level.

THERMOMETER

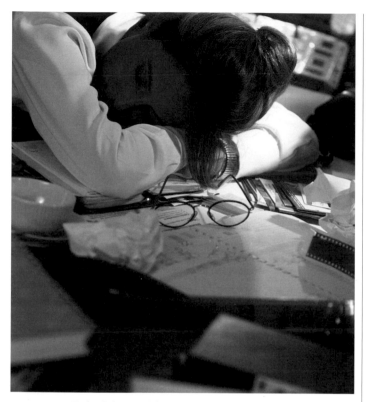

ABOVE *Feeling lethargic and sleepy maybe a sign of an underactive thyroid.*

HELPFUL FOODS
AND SUPPLEMENTS
FOR THE THYROID

People with an overactive thyroid have increased demands for many nutrients, and the B complex is particularly important since these vitamins are intimately involved with the release of energy from food. Wholegrains such as brown rice, seeds, fermented foods like miso paste (from soy), and yeast extract (if there is no allergy) are particularly good sources of B vitamins. Vitamin C from fruits and vegetables, vitamin E from olive oil and wholegrains, and essential fatty acids from seeds and fish are all required optimally in hyperthyroidism (an overactive thyroid).

Calcium from seeds, pulses (legumes), tofu, leafy green vegetables, and the soft bones of canned fish is especially important to thyroid sufferers (of either under- or overfunctioning) for reducing the risk of osteoporosis, regulation of heart beat, helping metabolize iron, and aiding in the transmission of nervous impulses. Magnesium from green leafy vegetables, wholegrains, beans, wheatgerm, figs, dried apricots, seeds, buckwheat, and fish is vital to help balance calcium levels, and in promoting a healthy cardiovascular system.

DO YOU SUFFER FROM AN OVERACTIVE THYROID?

A further set of questions to establish the possibility of an overactive thyroid (hyperthyroidism). Again, a simple "yes" or "no" answer is required

- Does your heart race and beat strongly even when you are resting?
- Is your pulse rate above 80 per minute when you are resting?
- Do you blush or have hot flashes?
- Do you have night sweats?
- Are you highly emotional, nervous, or irritable?
- Do you have twitches around the eyes or in the facial muscles?
- Do you suffer from insomnia?
- Are you aware of an inner trembling?
- Is your skin frequently moist (especially your palms)?
- Are you oversensitive to heat?
- Do your thoughts race and prevent clear thinking?
- Has your appetite increased, yet you are still not gaining weight?
- Have you started to get more menstrual problems?
- Has your sex drive increased?
- Have you eye or sight problems?
- Is there a swelling in your neck?
- Have your muscles lost their strength?
- Have you got blood pressure problems?

SCORING

Score one point for each "yes" answer.

If you have answered "yes" to half or more of these questions, carry out the basal temperature test, and visit your physician for a check up.

Manganese from nuts, wholegrains, and black tea helps those with an underactive thyroid (hypothyroidism). It is involved in the formation of the thyroid hormone, thyroxine, and can help eliminate fatigue, improve muscle function, aid memory, and reduce nervous irritability. Similarly, iodine is a mineral that forms part of the thyroxine molecule, and since this mineral is found in seaweeds (especially kelp), supplementing the diet with kelp extract is likely to help those with hypothyroidism. Thyroxine must be converted to its active form, known as tri-iodothyronine, before it can act; and for this conversion the minerals zinc, copper, and iron are required by the body.

Having an efficient metabolism is at the core of thyroid treatment. For our body chemistry to work well, the body's enzymes must be supplied with all the micronutrients necessary to work as co-factors. The minerals zinc, selenium, and magnesium are very important in this respect.

There is an increased requirement for vitamin A, as retinol, since beta-carotene is not easily converted to retinol by

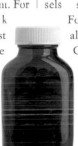

ABOVE
Manganese aids in the production of thyroxine.

the liver of thyroid sufferers. Attempting to obtain good levels of this vitamin from high intakes of beta-carotene does not work. Care must be taken with any foods (e.g. liver) or supplements containing vitamin A (as retinol) if pregnant or breastfeeding, since this form can soon become toxic.

ABOVE *Shellfish help to nourish and rebalance the thyroid gland.*

Some foods contain substances called goitrogens, which interfere with the workings of the thyroid gland. These substances occur naturally in several plants, particularly those belonging to the family *Cruciferae,* such as white turnip, cabbage, broccoli, cauliflower, Brussels sprouts, and mustard. Fortunately, cooking will usually inactivate goitrogens. Goitrogenic foods should, therefore, be used sparingly, or at least not eaten raw, by anyone with a thyroid complaint.

In addition to any medical care given to you by your physician, the best way to nourish your thyroid gland and enable it to rebalance is to undertake

the New Pyramid program, making sure that you eat fish, shellfish, and seaweed regularly, along with foods that are high in the antioxidants zinc, beta-carotene, vitamin C, and selenium (see pages 34–37).

Supplement complexes specifically designed for nourishing the thyroid gland include nutrients such as calcium, magnesium, selenium, zinc, vitamin A, vitamin C, niacinamide, and other B-complex vitamins, Siberian ginseng, kelp, licorice, and possibly the amino acids L-glycine, L-glutamine, and L-tyrosine. However, take extra care with kelp supplements or any food containing iodine, as an excess of this mineral will interfere greatly with thyroid function and could cause further imbalance. Ask for advise at your health food store if you are considering using kelp supplements.

BELOW
Seaweed contains iodine, good for those with hypothyroidism.

ABOVE *Oily fish is an essential part of the diet program for those with thyroid malfunction.*

Metabolism

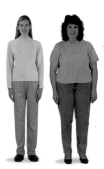

ABOVE *Some people don't put on weight however much they eat, while others put it on easily.*

MOST OF THE *amino acids, fats, and sugars in the bloodstream are transported to the liver after absorption from the intestines. Some nutrients go directly into the circulation and are delivered to all cells of the body, and others remain in the liver. Amino acids are reconstituted to make proteins, which are incorporated into the structure of the cells or become active molecules such as enzymes and antibodies. Excess protein is broken down and used to supply energy. Fats are also incorporated into the cell structure, and used as the basis for some hormones, for energy,or put into storage. Carbohydrates are mainly used to make energy.*

The utilization of these nutrients is called metabolism, and it occurs in every cell of the body. The chemical reactions involved in metabolism themselves require nutrients in the form of many different vitamins and minerals. Metabolism can be divided up into two parts – breakdown of nutrients (to release energy), and synthesis of new structures (to build new cells). The process of turning food into energy (breakdown) is called catabolism. Our cells oxidize carbohydrates, fatty acids, and excess amino acids to release energy. This energy is used to power the chemical processes that sustain life. Some of the energy released is used to help build new cells.

This process of building up nutrients to form new structures and new cells (biosynthesis) is called anabolism. The two processes – catabolism and anabolism – work together to keep the body functioning in accordance with information that is received from the genetic makeup of the cell. When the rate of one exceeds the rate of the other, health problems arise, the first of which is usually a change in body weight. Since a change to a lower metabolic rate is much more common than a move to a higher rate, overweight and obesity are seen as prime indicators in metabolic disharmony.

BY FAILING TO BREATHE PROPERLY MOST OF US SIMPLY DO NOT GET ENOUGH OXYGEN INTO OUR LUNGS

GOOD BREATHING IMPROVES THE EFFICIENCY OF THE METABOLISM

The daily requirement for energy varies depending on genes, gender, level of activity, state of health, and other factors, but on average, we probably need around 2,500 calories (really kilocalories) or 10,500 kJ (kilojoules). Part of this energy is used up by the body in maintaining normal processes, such as heartbeat and breathing, and our body will need this energy to satisfy this requirement whatever we are doing. This is the Basal Metabolic Rate.

LEFT *Many yoga techniques, such as the Cobra position shown here, are designed to improve the practice and efficiency of breathing.*

CORRECT MOVEMENT OF THE DIAPHRAGM IS THE KEY TO GOOD BREATHING

Some people have a naturally low basal metabolic rate, and tend to put on weight easily. Others have a high rate, and seem to be able to eat all the time and stay thin.

METABOLISM-BOOSTING FOODS

The best way of raising the metabolic rate is to eat a metabolism-boosting diet containing lots of fresh whole foods. Since carbohydrates are the principal energy-giving foods, you may feel that if you increase the amount of these you will obtain more energy and stimulate metabolism. However, to metabolize carbohydrate efficiently we need a host of different enzymes, and these depend on many different vitamins and minerals to act as co-factors. The important vitamins are the B complex, folic acid, and biotin, and the best sources are fresh fruit, raw vegetables, and wheatgerm. Seeds, nuts, and wholegrains also have reasonable levels. The minerals iron, calcium, magnesium, chromium, and zinc (all found in whole grains, seeds, and nuts) are vital for the manufacture of energy within the cells.

GETTING MORE OXYGEN

In addition to eating the wrong kinds of food, many people do not get enough oxygen into their lungs and bodies to maximize their energy levels. The biggest problem is incorrect breathing, or not breathing deeply enough (using only the upper part of the lungs), so that the total lung volume available is never approached. The modern lifestyle in the Western world is much to blame for this – sitting at desks most of the working day, driving to and from work or during leisure hours, and flopping in front of the television most evenings. If you interrupt your sedentary occupations regularly by carrying out a deep breathing routine, you will keep your mental and physical energy at a higher level.

You could start attending yoga classes, where correct deep breathing routines (called pranayamas) are an integral part of the practice; the postures also open the chest. The Alexander Technique will also help.

SMOKING

Smoking is the worst thing you can do to your oxygen levels, and therefore, your metabolism. Chemicals in tobacco smoke will damage the delicate lining of the lungs and prevent proper uptake of oxygen. They also enter the bloodstream, and cause many diseases.

Some of the chemicals in tobacco have a stimulating effect and will raise metabolism slightly, but there is a much healthier way. If you smoke, remember that you are not only damaging your body, but interfering with your body's capacity to produce energy as well.

TESTING YOUR METABOLIC RATE

Answer "yes" or "no" to the following.

● Do you have less energy, or become tired more easily, than friends of similar age and lifestyle to yourself?
● Do you seem to feel the cold more than most of the people in your family or group of friends?
● Do you find that you only have to eat very little extra food to start gaining weight?
● Have you recently been on a very low-calorie diet or a very low-carbohydrate diet, or have you taken slimming pills, such as amphetamines?
● Have you been on a calorie-restricted diet continuously over the last six months or longer?
● Do you have weak and/or poorly defined muscles?
● Is your hair thinning?
● Do your ankles swell, particularly at night?

SCORING

Score one point for each "yes" answer.

0 – 3 You are unlikely to have a slow metabolism.
4– 5 Your metabolism is on the low side, but after a few weeks on the New Pyramid program you will find your energy levels rising, and any excess weight disappearing.
6 and over You have quite a low metabolic rate and have the type of metabolism that responds quickly to food being in short supply. If you have been trying to lose weight for a long time, you may have reduced lean tissue and laid down more fat. The New Pyramid program is ideal for you, but try to obtain carbohydrate from vegetables and pulses (legumes) instead of grains.

IMPROVING METABOLISM WITH ACTIVITY AND EXERCISE

When you reach the stage where you are beginning to feel the benefits of a healthy metabolism-boosting program (a good wholefood diet, and improved breathing), the next natural step is to look for ways of being more active. As your energy levels rise, your body begins to feel more alive. Life becomes more interesting and you want to dive into things. If you are a hardworking person with a job and family to look after, finding time to undertake additional activities may seem a daunting prospect. However, when your metabolic fires are truly burning brighter, you will begin to have much more than just a passing urge to do things and will find that you make the time.

Use the increased energy that is pushing for an outlet to enhance metabolism, and do it in a way that both fits in with your daily routine (run upstairs, run for a bus, walk to work, cycle to work, dance around with the vacuum cleaner, walk briskly with the baby carriage or buggy), and in ways that will interest you; scan the local press, night-school class prospectuses, gym and leisure center advertisements to find an activity that you would really like to take part in two or three times a week.

Many people who try to lose weight and improve health by exercise alone, or by a combination of diet and exercise, fail because they do not understand the metabolic processes involved. When we begin to exercise, muscle tissue uses its

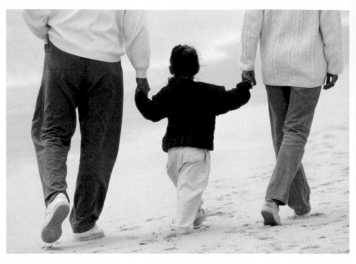

ABOVE *You don't need a gym or running shoes; regular walking is good exercise.*

local supply of glycogen, and there is a delay before any fat is mobilized or more glycogen is released from the liver. This is why warming up is so important; it helps to get this process started. Most beginners do not continue exercising for long enough to break through the warm-up barrier, and they tend to give up as their muscle glycogen stores begin to run out – just at the time when they are about to start burning any excess body fat. If you never exercise continuously for more than a few minutes, your fat reserves won't diminish and stamina won't improve. The more this happens, the more the muscles will rely on their own stores of glycogen and the less readily they will burn fat. However, after about 10 to 20 minutes of continuous, moderate exercise, fat becomes an increasingly important source of muscle fuel, and the metabolism becomes more efficient.

You do not need to start running marathons. The fact is that brisk walking in the fresh air, or even on a treadmill in a gym, is by far the best way to start. The longer the activity continues, the greater the proportion of fat that will be used as fuel and the fitter you will become. As you begin to exercise regularly, the faster will be the switch from pure glycogen to the glycogen/fat mixture. The more you exercise the faster the oxygen will move to the tissues, as your heart and lungs become better conditioned.

The more active you are, the more excess fat you will shed, and the healthier and fitter you will be. Eventually you will reach a stable point where food, activity, and your whole lifestyle are in balance and at a level that is right for you. As you get used to using your body for an increased level of energy output, so your capacity for pleasure will grow. This is called positive feedback. The more you do, the more you will be able to do and the more you will want to do.

BALANCING HORMONES NATURALLY

Finally, in addition to these changes your body will also begin to undergo a balancing of hormones. Our hormones, like every other part of our unique selves, have a specific profile. The hormone profile of an unfit overweight person is different from that of a healthy slim person. With the rebalancing of your hormones, your transition will be complete. A rebalancing of your hormones will not change your sexuality. You are likely to find, however, that one of the rewards of a slim, active, healthy body is a greatly enhanced capacity for sensual and sexual satisfaction. Sex is improved by the correct balance of our hormonal system. Unfit, unhealthy, overweight people have lost their balance and will find that some of the spice has gone out of life.

Hormones are intimately involved with the metabolism of fat. Growth hormone, made in the pituitary gland, is a liberator of fat from the fat stores of the body. Being active causes a rise in the level of this hormone; it increases sharply at about 10 to 15 minutes into a vigorous exercise period. If you are an adult, growth hormone will not actually increase your size (though it has this effect on children), but it will promote the growth of lean tissue within your body, provided you are eating enough of the right sorts of foods.

Once you become more physically active, other hormone changes occur. Muscular effort, combined with the excitement of doing something you really enjoy, leads to the production of adrenaline and noradrenaline from the adrenal glands. These hormones make you feel active and energetic and they reduce appetite. Insulin (from the pancreas) is another hormone important in fat metabolism. As activity is increased, the production of insulin decreases. Since insulin is involved in fat storage, anything that balances the levels of insulin will prevent fat deposition. The combined effects of regular exercise and the New Pyramid program will enhance metabolism and reduce the tendency to store excess body fat, while encouraging the muscles to burn fat.

BELOW *A depressed metabolism can lead to overtiredness.*

BELOW *A healthy metabolism improves vigor and energy.*

AWARENESS OF BEING OVERWEIGHT CAN MAKE YOU UNHAPPY

A VIGOROUS APPROACH TO LIFE

CIRCULATION IS POORER AND HORMONES UNBALANCED

WELL DEVELOPED MUSCLES

GOOD CIRCULATION AND BALANCED HORMONES

TAUT ABDOMEN

LIMBS BECOME TIRED MORE EASILY

POOR MUSCLE TONE

ENERGETIC LIMBS

71

Weight Gain and Health

BEING OVERWEIGHT *can be dangerous to health. Research indicates that at present more than a quarter of the population of Britain is classed as overweight – 37 percent of men and 24 percent of women. Of these, some are obese, which is defined as being more than 20 percent above your ideal weight. American research has shown a steep rise in the numbers of overweight adults from a quarter of the population between 1960 and 1980, to a third of the population between 1980 and 1991 – a 32 percent increase in 10 years. Results from a U.S. government study show that young adults (25 to 30) are getting fatter fastest of all, and that more than 20 percent of the U.S. population are clinically obese.*

LEFT *Measuring the proportion of your waist to hips will tell you what body type you are.*

MEASURING EXCESS WEIGHT

As a general rule of thumb, a B.M.I. (body mass index) between 20 and 28 is seen as normal, and anything over 28 as overweight. B.M.I.s over 30 are seriously overweight, with anything over B.M.I. 40 classified as obese. A B.M.I. under 20 can be regarded as underweight. The calculation disregards age and gender considerations, and avoids making a judgment about large or small frames.

FAT DISTRIBUTION

A further complication is the distribution of fat. Android type obesity (fat on the upper body and within the abdomen) is more commonly associated with cardiovascular disease and diabetes than is the gynoid pattern (fat on the buttocks and thighs). As a guide to determine which type you are, the waist/hip circumference for women should not exceed 0.8, or 1.0 for men, regardless of the individual's B.M.I.

CALCULATING YOUR BODY MASS INDEX

A simple calculation can be used to give you some idea of the dividing line between underweight, normal weight, and overweight.

It is called the Body Mass Index and is calculated as follows:

$$\frac{\text{weight in kilograms}}{\text{height in meters, squared}} = \text{B.M.I.}$$

For example, for a woman 5ft 2in tall and weighing 168 pounds, we would have the calculation:

168 pounds ÷ 2.25 = around 75 kg
(Divide by 2.25 to give kilograms)
5ft 2in is 62 inches
62 x 0.0254 = 1.58 meters
(Multiply by 0.0254 to give meters)
This figure has to be squared
1.58 x 1.58 = 2.5

The final calculation of B.M.I. is:
$$\frac{75}{2.5} = 30$$
A B.M.I. of 30 would suggest that the woman in this example is overweight.

For example, if a woman has a waist measurement of 30 inches (76cm) and a hip measurement of 36 inches (92cm), then the calculation of: 30/36 = 0.83 shows us that this woman has more fat accumulated around the waist than is healthy, and is a rather large "apple".

Although we are genetically "programed" to have either an "apple" (android) or a "pear" (gynoid) shape, good nutrition and a little exercise will go a long way to removing the extra risk of ill health that is associated with being an "apple".

Despite there being more overweight men than women, twice as many women as men are trying to lose weight. Of these women, around 17 percent are trying to shrink below a healthy weight. This is a very bad state of affairs for the women concerned but not for the diet food industry.

However, for those individuals who are truly overweight to the point of obesity there is a substantial risk to their health from a number of diseases, such as cardiovascular disease, cancer, and diabetes. American estimates indicate that the cost of treating conditions relating to obesity in 1986 was $39 billion. Problems of self-image may seem unimportant from a health point of view, but they nevertheless cause much misery and lowering of self-esteem, which can have a disastrous effect on social life, work, and relationships; this, in turn, has an effect on our health.

It is women who, on the whole, suffer from a poor self-image. The stereotype of the slim female is now thought to be the reason why more teenage girls are taking up smoking and using amphetamines in an attempt to "look cool", raise metabolism, and stave off hunger pangs.

ACHIEVING A HEALTHY BODY WEIGHT

The conclusion to be drawn about achieving a healthy body weight and shape can be summed up as follows.

❁ Aim for a B.M.I. of between 20 and 28 (no more or less) by using a metabolism-boosting diet such as the New Pyramid program.
❁ Aim to reduce fat accumulation around the waist by good nutrition and exercise.
❁ Avoid smoking, amphetamines or diet pills, and the excessive use of stimulant beverages.
❁ Attempt to find other ways of improving your self-image while you are losing weight, such as having a new hairstyle or pampering yourself.

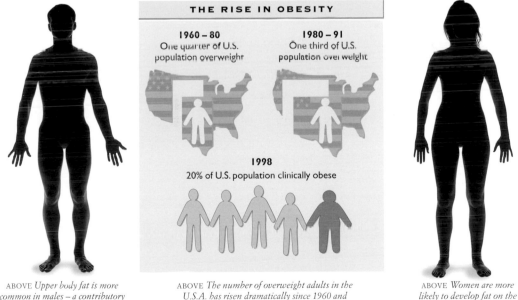

THE RISE IN OBESITY

1960 – 80
One quarter of U.S. population overweight

1980 – 91
One third of U.S. population overweight

1998
20% of U.S. population clinically obese

ABOVE *Upper body fat is more common in males – a contributory factor to heart disease.*

ABOVE *The number of overweight adults in the U.S.A. has risen dramatically since 1960 and continues to rise today.*

ABOVE *Women are more likely to develop fat on the thighs than the upper body.*

WHY DO WE GET FAT?

Apart from any psychological reason, what biochemical changes cause us to become overweight in the first place? Why does it happen more particularly in later years? Why is it so hard to lose this weight?

Of course, we all know that the extra weight is due to extra fat (unless we are into excessive body building) and this has obviously accumulated by eating more food than we are metabolizing. For years we have been spoonfed the notion that "energy in" must always equal "energy out" or our weight will change. We can now see that there is a middle component to the equation that is rarely mentioned, giving us a more complicated formula: energy in (food) – basic body functions (or basal metabolism) = energy out (or muscular activity). This shows that losing weight is not a simple matter of "burning it off"; it also shows that we can control our weight much more effectively if we consume foods that allow for the nature of our basal metabolism.

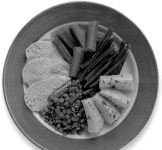

ABOVE *Choosing healthy food will help control weight, whatever the other relevant factors.*

Most diets concentrate on ways of consuming fewer energy units – such as low-fat diets, crash diets, liquid diets, meal replacement diets, mono diets (eating only one food type), high-fiber diets – while others include foods that are believed to be harder to digest, examples of these being high-protein diets, and starch/fat blocker diets. Some further types of diet concentrate on "special herbs or vegetables". Few diets have been designed to stimulate and balance the metabolism.

Furthermore, food allergy has been particularly implicated where individuals have found it very difficult to lose weight. Food allergies are likely to depress metabolism by

THE BRAIN BOTH RECEIVES AND TRANSMITS MESSAGES THROUGH THE NERVES

THE SPINAL CORD AND BRAIN CONSTITUTE THE CENTRAL NERVOUS SYSTEM

THE BRAIN CONTROLS THE MUSCLES THROUGH NERVES

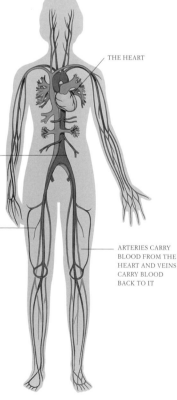

THE HEART

THE AORTA IS THE MAIN OUTFLOW ARTERY FROM THE HEART

THE BODY IS FULL OF TINY BLOOD VESSELS CALLED CAPILLARIES

ARTERIES CARRY BLOOD FROM THE HEART AND VEINS CARRY BLOOD BACK TO IT

LEFT AND RIGHT *The functioning of the body systems, such as the nervous and circulatory systems, affects weight.*

having a negative effect on the activity of the thyroid gland. By avoiding the major food allergens (wheat, dairy foods, citrus fruit, yeast, etc.) you are likely to improve the activity level of your metabolism and lose weight. A more accurate assessment of food allergy is now available, which tests samples of an individual's blood against a range of foods to assess any reaction.

Unfortunately, one of the problems with diets that reduce calorie intake below 1,000 per day is that the body sees this lowered amount of food as a threat of famine and it takes action by slowing down the metabolic rate by as much as 40 percent! At this point, you need less food than you did before just to maintain your weight at the same level. When you have been on one of these very low-calorie diets for a time, the minute you return to "normal" eating, the weight piles back on even faster than before.

A metabolically stimulating diet (such as the New Pyramid program), fulfills all five criteria of a healthy weight-loss diet:
• it produces weight loss;
• it is good for your health;
• it educates you in a healthy way of eating for your whole life;
• it is relatively easy to carry out;
• it doesn't leave you hungry, lethargic, or exhausted.

CALORIFIC CHART

This chart provides a guide to how many calories per minute are expended on each activity.

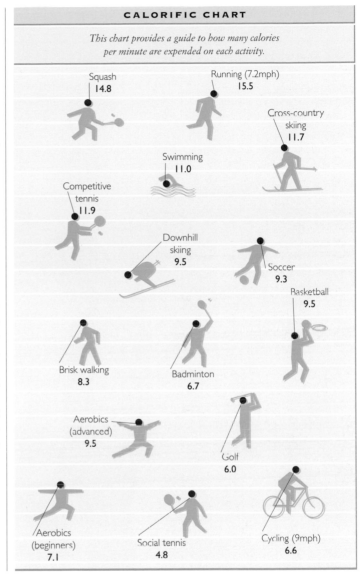

Squash 14.8

Running (7.2mph) 15.5

Cross-country skiing 11.7

Swimming 11.0

Competitive tennis 11.9

Downhill skiing 9.5

Soccer 9.3

Basketball 9.5

Brisk walking 8.3

Badminton 6.7

Aerobics (advanced) 9.5

Golf 6.0

Aerobics (beginners) 7.1

Social tennis 4.8

Cycling (9mph) 6.6

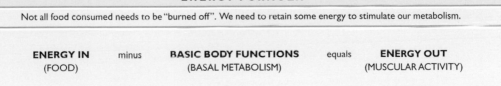

ENERGY FORMULA

Not all food consumed needs to be "burned off". We need to retain some energy to stimulate our metabolism.

ENERGY IN (FOOD)	minus	**BASIC BODY FUNCTIONS** (BASAL METABOLISM)	equals	**ENERGY OUT** (MUSCULAR ACTIVITY)

THE FAT CONNECTION

Some quick-fix diets lead us to believe that our bodies can actually lose 7 pounds (about 3kg) of fat in a week. This is ludicrous. The maximum, in normal circumstances, is more like 2 pounds a week, but 1 pound is more realistic. Any more than this is likely to be water, which will easily return, or muscle tissue, which would be disastrous. Since a large amount of energy is expended on lean tissue metabolism, losing any of this will quickly reduce basal metabolic rate.

Since fat is the most energy-dense (high calorific content) food group, many diets are based on reducing fat intake. Nevertheless, essential fatty acids must still be part of our healthy eating program. There is no need for saturated fats in any diet, but certain polyunsaturated fats, such as those found in fish, nuts, and seeds and seed oils, are essential to optimum health.

Apart from the problems with saturated fat itself, there are the unnatural substances that occur frequently in processed fats, primarily in margarines, shortenings (and, therefore, in cakes, pastries, and cookies), chips, and confectionery (especially chocolate). These substances are the hydrogenated oils and trans-fatty acids that will interfere with efficient metabolism and will slow weight loss considerably. They must be avoided at all costs.

Most of the fat in the average diet comes from meat, dairy produce, margarines and spreads, and high-fat processed or "fast" foods, so all of these foods need either to be kept to a very low level or eliminated.

THE CALORIE CONNECTION

Most nutrition books tell us that if you take what you eat and deduct what you burn off through exercise, the remainder ends up as flab round your middle; so, if you want to lose weight, you should eat less or exercise more, or both.

This theory just doesn't work. For example, a slice of wholewheat bread contains around 100 calories and if you made sure that you omitted one slice of wholewheat bread

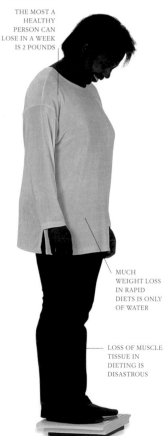

THE MOST A HEALTHY PERSON CAN LOSE IN A WEEK IS 2 POUNDS

MUCH WEIGHT LOSS IN RAPID DIETS IS ONLY OF WATER

LOSS OF MUSCLE TISSUE IN DIETING IS DISASTROUS

ABOVE *Quick-fix diets reduce weight, but in such a way that it soon returns afterward.*

every day then over at year you would, theoretically, have lost 36,500 calories. If we take it that 1 pound (0.45kg) of fat is just over 4,000 calories, in that first year you should have lost around 9 pounds of fat. All simply by not eating one slice of bread per day! Of course, this simply doesn't happen. The reason why this "calorie theory" does not add up is because it does not take into account metabolism, or any psychological or physiological problems associated with weight gain. Our metabolism has the job of turning the energy units in food into energy. People vary considerably in their ability to do this, and unlucky people with slow metabolisms will inevitably turn more food into fat.

THE CARBOHYDRATE CONNECTION

The body is designed to work properly on complex carbohydrates (carbohydrates that release their sugar units slowly) such as vegetables, lentils, beans, wholegrains and fruit. These foods, when properly digested, produce a more consistent level of energy, especially when correctly balanced with protein and fat, preventing the lows and highs of blood sugar that produce our bad moods, our ravenous hunger, and the temptation to binge on the nearest morsel.

When our blood-sugar levels are more stable, our energy levels are more balanced and we have longer relief from hunger. All of these factors will give the body a better chance to use up and metabolize the food properly rather than simply turning it into fat.

METABOLISM AND FAT LOSS

Metabolism is adaptive. When food intake is moderate and constant, fat accumulation occurs only when muscle mass is small. But when food intake is reduced, metabolic processes adjust to the new input level.

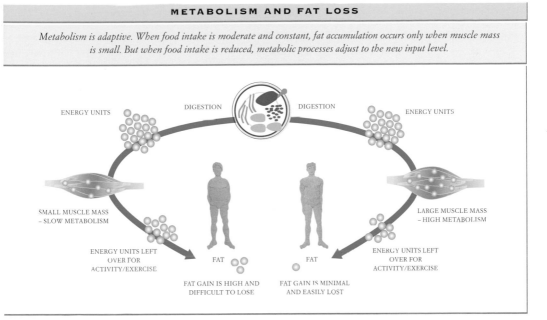

ENERGY UNITS   DIGESTION   DIGESTION   ENERGY UNITS

SMALL MUSCLE MASS – SLOW METABOLISM

LARGE MUSCLE MASS – HIGH METABOLISM

ENERGY UNITS LEFT OVER FOR ACTIVITY/EXERCISE   FAT   FAT   ENERGY UNITS LEFT OVER FOR ACTIVITY/EXERCISE

FAT GAIN IS HIGH AND DIFFICULT TO LOSE

FAT GAIN IS MINIMAL AND EASILY LOST

THE CORRECT MACRONUTRIENT BALANCE

In Britain, it would appear that the average diet derives approximately 44 percent of energy units (calories) from fat, 15 percent from protein and the remaining 41 percent from carbohydrates (usually of the refined white and sugary types). In the U.S.A., the average diet derives more than all 48 percent of energy in units from fat, and roughly 26 percent each from proteins and carbohydrates; in both countries too much fat is consumed.

Modern nutritional research suggests that the ideal diet should derive no more than 30 percent of calories from fat, 30 percent from protein, and the remaining 40 percent from complex carbohydrates. These new figures complement exactly what has been outlined in the New Pyramid progam. slow-release, complex carbohydrates, and their relationship to protein and fat. This balance is important for sustained energy, and the prevention of peaks and troughs of blood sugar. If we convert these caloritic percentages to actual amounts of food, we arrive at the ratio of 4:3 carbohydrate to protein (since they supply almost the same amount of energy gram for gram). We can then add on the ratio of 1.5 for total fat. (This is a low amount since fat supplies around twice as much energy per gram as either carbohydrate or protein.)

The overall ratio is then 4:3:1.5 (or 8:6:3) carbohydrate: protein: fat. As has been explained, the best types of carbohydrate are vegetables, lentils, beans, fruit, and whole grains, and not pasta, bread, and potatoes. The best (easily absorbable) protein is obtained from fish, poultry, tofu, seeds, and nuts. The best types of fats are those containing mono unsaturated fatty acids, such as olive oil and polyunsaturated fatty acids, which are found in fish, seeds, and nuts.

BELOW *The body works best on complex carbohydrates, such as vegetables, pulses, nuts, and wholegrains.*

THE FIBER CONNECTION

It was back in the 1980s that the F-Plan Diet, by Audrey Eyton, was first published and appeared to be a major solution to the hunger problems caused by low-calorie diets.

Adding fiber to the diet helps you to feel full for longer and hence reduces appetite, as well as having other health benefits. We know that a diet containing 1 ounce (27g) of fiber daily will prevent constipation and help prevent more severe forms of bowel problems such as diverticular disease. A diet high in natural fiber will also prevent reabsorption of toxins and cholesterol.

"High fiber" does not mean piling mountains of wheat or other bran onto our food. The correct way to a high fiber diet is to include lots of fiber-rich vegetables, pulses (legumes), and fruit, and some wholegrains in our diet. The fiber in vegetables, fruit, lentils, beans, and oats is much more gentle and effective. Fiber not only makes you feel full for longer, it also helps to control blood-sugar levels, by releasing sugar into the blood slowly and over a longer length of time.

THE PROTEIN CONNECTION

When consumed in excess, protein is broken down to release sugar-like molecules that can be used as fuel. Otherwise, proteins would have no calorific value in energy tables. Protein has only half the calories of fat and requires more energy for its digestion than carbohydrates or fat. For these two reasons, protein would seem the ideal material for dieters. However, very high unlimited protein diets put the liver and kidneys under stress and make the body more acidic.

Protein is needed for building new tissues in a growing child, and for replacing and repairing worn out and damaged tissues in everyone, but it is only needed in moderation. As a rough guide, if we are of average size and sedentary, we probably need around 7 ounces (180g) of protein-rich food, such as fish, poultry, lean meat, cottage cheese, or tofu, a day. If we are above average in size (taller or fatter), or take vigorous exercise daily, we are likely to require as much as 12 ounces (320g) of protein-rich food.

BELOW *Protein is essential to both children and adults, as it provides the body's building blocks.*

THE BRAIN NEEDS PROTEIN AS MUCH AS THE REST OF THE BODY

BODY TISSUE IS BUILT FROM AMINO ACIDS, WHICH ARE DERIVED FROM PROTEIN

PROTEIN IS ESSENTIAL FOR GROWTH

THE MICRONUTRIENT CONNECTION

The ability of your body to burn fat does not depend solely on the types and amounts of carbohydrate, fat, and protein in your diet. It also depends on the activity of vitamins and minerals that are consumed. These micronutrients are essential in controlling the breakdown of glucose, and other digestive end products, which in turn releases energy, together with other biochemical substances, to all our body cells. Any lack of these micronutrients will result in lowered physical energy and, theoretically, a tendency for the tired body to lay down fat.

The transport of glucose from the blood into the cells depends upon the presence of vitamins B_3 and B_6, and the minerals chromium and zinc. The actual breakdown of glucose within the cells into energy requires vitamins B_1, B_2, B_3, B_5, C, and the mineral iron. Another substance called coenzyme Q10 is also required. Magnesium is required for A.T.P. (energy) production. Insuring an adequate supply of these nutrients is theoretically going to increase the effectiveness of any weight-loss program. It is always preferable to obtain micronutrients from food, but in some cases, especially if your digestion is a little under par, or if you suffer from food intolerances, supplementing your diet with mineral and vitamin preparations may be required, at least for a while.

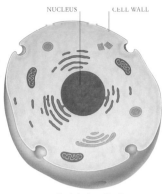

NUCLEUS   CELL WALL

ABOVE *Each body cell relies on micronutrients – vitamins and minerals – to process the fuel it needs.*

The release of energy from cells is also helped by the activity of the minerals iron, calcium, magnesium chromium, and zinc, which are generally deficient in the Western diet. In all, 22 vitamins, and minerals are needed for proper metabolism and weight control. The ten most important are vitamins B_1, B_2, B_3, B_5, B_6, C, choline and inositol, and minerals magnesium, chromium and zinc.

EXERCISE

To remove excess fat effectively, we need to increase our level of activity and so increase energy output. Exercise also tones up our muscles so that as we lose weight, our new skin fits nicely instead of sagging.

Exercise on its own, without dieting, doesn't actually help to promote much weight loss; only around 300 calories are burned up by running a mile! But the effects of consistent exercise are cumulative. So, it is the frequency of exercise, not the intensity, that is important.

As weight is lost and muscle is built up with exercise, the body will need more oxygen to allow extra muscle tissue to work efficiently.

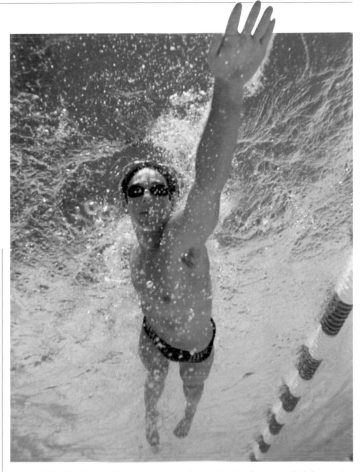

ABOVE *After 20 minutes of aerobic exercise, such as swimming, fat starts to fuel the muscles.*

The best kind of exercise is, therefore, aerobic. Continuous exercise such as swimming, jogging, brisk walking, or cycling are more aerobic than "stop-go" exercises such as tennis or squash. Playing tennis uses more of the "fast" muscle fibers that use glucose for fuel. You will lose weight playing tennis or squash but it will require you to play for a very long time compared to the time spent swimming, cycling, running, or walking. Since the amount of fat you carry is a far more important statistic than your weight, don't use your scales as the only means of monitoring progress; encouragement in the early days is likely to come from a reduction in "vital statistics" rather than loss of weight. As you start to exercise aerobically, you will begin to replace fatty tissue with lean muscle.

In addition, contrary to popular belief, moderate exercise decreases your appetite by encouraging the appetite mechanism to work properly. Exercise also releases brain chemicals called endorphins, which give you a sense of well-being.

CALORIE COUNTING

The number of energy units in a food (calories) varies according to the food group. This knowledge has triggered a large amount of laboratory analysis of a wide range of foods (calorimetry), and out of this work "calorie guides" have been produced. The diet methods that rely on calorie counting depend upon these tables.

The main problems with calorie counting include the sheer amount of effort that has to be put in to calculate how many calories there are in any one of your meals, from the weighing to the mathematics. But by far the most important problem is that, because the usual limit is around 1,000 calories per day, these diets are very hard to stick to; hunger pangs are never far away.

Also, the mathematics of calorie counting if taken to their full extent produce some very spurious results. As we have seen, by the omission of an item of food each day (such as sliced bread), at the end of a year we will have a useful 9 pound (4.05kg) loss. But there is no way that simply omitting one slice of bread a day will result in a loss of 46 pounds (20.25kg) after 5 years and 91 pounds (40.5kg) after 10 years. Clearly calorie-counting, though it works in the short term, pays no attention to metabolism, and is, therefore, ultimately ineffective.

VERY LOW-CALORIE DIETS

These are the liquid or "milkshake" diets. Their aim is to severely cut daily calorie intake, sometimes to as low as 400Kcals (calories) for women and 500Kcals for men, but at the same time provide at least the recommended daily allowances (R.D.A.s) of major vitamins and minerals. These "shakes" provide around 40g of protein for women and 50g for men. The addition of protein allows some prevention of the breakdown of muscle tissue to produce energy. Weight is definitely lost on these regimes, and the high level of micronutrients in the product is probably the reason for the sense of well-being that is often encountered within the first week or so of these diets.

However, with such a low daily calorific intake, it is certain that lean muscle tissue, in addition to fat, will be lost from the body. This type of "crash dieting" also lowers metabolic rate, and since a very small intake of normal food will encourage the weight to return, the long-term results are likely to be unsatisfactory.

HIGH-FIBER DIETS

If what you are looking for is bulky food to make you feel full while still reducing your calorie intake, then you may feel that this type of diet is for you. Fiber in its natural form, found in vegetables, fruit,

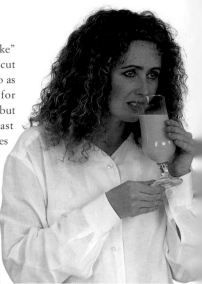

ABOVE *There are many low-calorie diet drinks on the market.*

nuts, seeds, and grains, absorbs water and gives the feeling of fullness for longer even though fewer calories may have been eaten. Additionally a high-fiber diet reduces the risk of bowel cancer, diabetes, or diverticular disease.

Fiber is also fairly free of calories and for all these reasons, it is easy to see why a low-calorie, high-fiber diet is easier to follow, healthier, and more satisfying to eat than low-calorie diets without fiber.

However, this type of regime produces fairly poor weight loss and, in some cases the diet produces an irritated colon since wheat fiber in particular is very rough on our insides. The other problem is that fiber not only helps to remove waste materials from the body, but also too much can leach out important micronutrients. You should insure that you obtain fiber from natural sources rather than from bran supplements.

LEFT *Simply omitting one slice of bread a day from your diet does not produce constant weight loss.*

HIGH-FAT/LOW-CARBOHYDRATE DIETS

People who advocate high-fat, low-carbohydrate diets believe that if you don't eat any carbohydrate foods, you must burn fat instead. However, trying to burn fat without some carbohydrate present is like trying to set fire to a lump of coal without using a firelighter.

A diet that is burning off only fat releases substances called ketones into the blood. High ketone levels in the blood are extremely dangerous and these substances must be removed quickly via the kidneys. Therefore, a high blood-ketone level puts the kidneys under stress.

Not only is a high-fat diet that is low in carbohydrates very difficult to produce and maintain, it causes ineffective metabolism and produces toxins – neither of which leads to healthy weight loss. In addition, your intake of hydrogenated fats and trans fatty acids is likely to be very high. To all these drawbacks are added the problems caused by saturated fats – clogged arteries and the risk of cardiovascular disease.

We do need some fat in the diet (essential fatty acids together with fat-soluble vitamins) but no-one can become healthier on a diet where fat is the major energy food.

RIGHT *Fiber, taken in its natural form in fiber-rich foods, produces a satisfying feeling of being full.*

HIGH-PROTEIN DIETS

Although this type of regime can be quite effective in the short term, consuming unlimited amounts of protein – even if it is lean meat, poultry, and fish, or even large amounts of pulses (legumes) – can have an unhealthy outcome.

Protein has only half the calories of the same amount of fat, and is harder to metabolize. It is argued that because protein is harder to convert to fuel, fewer calories are consumed by the body. Although this is true, there are other problems with high-protein diets: liver and kidney stress and increased tissue acidity which can lead to osteoporosis and arthritis.

ABOVE *Excess animal protein harms the liver and skeleton.*

Because protein is harder to digest, some proteins may not be digested completely before parts of them are absorbed into the bloodstream. We are then at greater risk from developing food intolerances, and, possibly, even auto-immune disease, such as rheumatoid arthritis.

A diet high in non-organic animal protein is likely to carry with it a cocktail of antibiotics and hormones, both of which will interfere with optimum metabolism. Eating a diet of excessive protein could affect our liver, kidneys, skeleton, and toxic levels adversely and may be responsible for the development of intolerances and allergies.

JUST ADDING BRAN TO FOOD CAN CREATE MINERAL DEFICIENCY

WHEAT FIBER CAN CAUSE AN IRRITATED COLON

STARCH-BLOCKER DIETS

This isn't so much a specific diet of certain foods, but rather a pill, taken before each meal, containing substances that will block the digestion and/or uptake of starch from our diets. The theory is that you can eat as much carbohydrate as you like without absorbing it.

Scientific analytical work undertaken on these "starch blockers" found no evidence of any effect on carbohydrate metabolism. Moreover, in addition to finding very variable levels of the starch inhibitor enzymes (which were supposed to be doing the blocking), a substance called lectin was found. This is a potentially dangerous material, though rendered harmless if cooked. It is found in beans (especially uncooked red kidney beans) from which the starch blocker pill is manufactured.

Taking these pills does nothing whatsoever to retrain the dieter in the ways of healthy eating, and may even cause toxicity. The most obvious result of diets using starch blockers is an increase in flatulence!

FUNCTIONS OF SOLUBLE FIBER GELS

❋ Maintaining digestive regularity (by allowing the efficient movement of food through the intestinal tract).
❋ Slowing the release of sugars into the blood (which is helpful for people suffering from non-insulin-dependent diabetes and hypoglycemia).
❋ Helping with some of the problems associated with irritable bowel and allergies.
❋ Improving intestinal conditions (by protecting the bowel lining and encouraging growth of bowel flora).
❋ Reducing cholesterol, triglycerides, and free fatty acids in the body.

Starch-blocker diets are not to be confused with the type of diets that use fiber supplements that are taken before meals as a means of curbing appetite before the next meal is eaten. Usually this involves taking encapsulated powdered fiber with a large glass of water 30 minutes before eating. The water then reacts with the fiber, making it swell and fill up part of the stomach. Several types of fibrous materials are used; they are usually of the soluble fiber type and are related to celluloses, pectins, and mucilages found in a range of plants. This form of diet is useful in the short term, but is not recommended as a long-term dietary lifestyle.

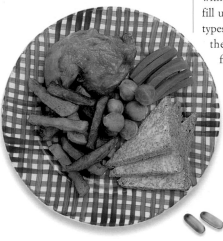

LEFT *Certain pills are designed to be taken with meals to stop the body absorbing carbohydrate.*

WATER-LOSS DIETS

Water-loss diets are simply ways of using freeze-dried and encapsulated diuretic herbs and vegetables, such as asparagus, to rid the body of water. No one is doubting for a minute that the herbs, vegetables, or other special foods, do the job of removing water, however, they do not burn fat, and may put an extra strain on the kidneys. Using these diets in the short term may be beneficial, but for long-lasting weight loss that insures a healthy way of life, they go no way to break old self-defeating patterns of eating or establishing new, more healthy, fat-burning ones.

Other techniques could be included under this heading, such as special clothing, body wraps, seaweed wraps, mud wraps, mineral baths, and saunas, all of which profess to rid the body of excess water and "impurities". Again, there is no doubt that they work in the short term, and, as they encourage sweating, a certain amount of waste material will be removed along with the water. You may feel wonderful after one of these treatments, but none of them are likely to do much about stored fat in the long term.

THE DIET OF THE CARBOHYDRATE-ADDICT

This way of eating is for those individuals who feel that they cannot stick to the usual low-calorie type of regime, simply because they love their carbohydrates (grains, cakes, candies, breads, etc.). What the exponents of this diet say is that is doesn't matter how much carbohydrate you eat, nor even what type of carbohydrate you consume (this

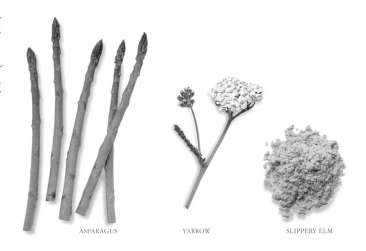

BROOM TOPS

ASPARAGUS

YARROW

SLIPPERY ELM

ABOVE *Water-loss diets use known diuretics, often freeze-dried herbs or vegetables such as these above.*

includes alcohol), as long as you only eat carbohydrate once a day within the period of about an hour before 8:00 p.m. Other meals are to be very low in carbohydrate or devoid of carbohydrate altogether, and are therefore comprised of fairly large amounts of protein and fat.

The theory behind this diet revolves around the excessive production of insulin that can sometimes occur in individuals who have consumed large and frequent amounts of refined carbohydrates over long periods of time. It is argued that this hyperinsulinemia (excessive insulin production and/or insulin insensitivity) is the cause of the unsatisfied hunger. After eating a meal containing carbohydrate improperly balanced with protein and fat, too much insulin is produced and some remains in the blood.

Most of this theory is very logical, but consuming a diet high in complex carbohydrates, well-balanced with protein, and omitting refined sugar and starch is a healthier way of controlling blood sugar and hunger.

THE LOW-FAT DIET

Many people have had a good deal of success on this type of diet, where you are able to eat lots of carbohydrate, mostly the complex type, and moderate protein, but fat is very restricted. Yet the "forbidden list" includes many natural wholefoods that are essential to dietary balance and providers of essential fatty acids and fat-soluble vitamins, such as seeds and seed oils, nuts, fatty fish, and avocados. The omission of these foods from the diet will, in the long term, cause havoc with the endocrine (hormonal) system and immune status.

People who eat very low-fat diets could be reducing their ability to fight infection. For example, recent investigation into blood samples from competitive marathon runners indicated that those who had been getting their energy from a 15 percent fat diet, as opposed to a more reasonable 30 percent,

had fewer infection-fighting white cells in their blood after exercise when compared to athletes on the higher-fat diet. In addition, research indicates that people with lower than normal blood-cholesterol levels are more prone to cancer.

BELOW *People on low-fat diets have fewer white blood cells, so run the risk of making themselves susceptible to infections*

WHY DIETING DOESN'T WORK

Conventional dieting regimes assume that if you reduce your input of food and go hungry, you will lose fat. National statistics have disproved this on a massive scale, since decade by decade we have been dieting more, yet on average, we weigh more. Looking at it another way, in the past 30 years or so there have been dozens of new miracle weight-loss diets that have been followed by millions of people; many of these diets also include exercise programs, yet very few dieters have reached their goal and maintained a healthy weight. Part of the problem stems from our unique biochemistry. Each person, as we know, has their own individual nutrient needs, and it is, therefore, impossible to set out a single simple diet that will guarantee success for everyone.

METABOLISM

It is very likely that one of the reasons for people becoming fatter is the basic problem of low or inefficient metabolism caused by either a low intake of the micronutrients needed to assist metabolic enzymes, and/or a high level of pollutants entering the body and causing a greater amount of energy to be channeled into removing these metabolism-blocking substances. In the calorie-counting process, a dieter on 1,000 calories a day from refined and processed food will have nowhere near the micronutrient and metabolism-boosting content of one on 1,000 calories from a diet wholegrains, fresh vegetables, fruits, lean meats, fish, seeds, nuts, and pulses (legumes). Both dieters may initially lose weight, but the wholefood dieter will be much healthier, more vital, and will be able to continue to lose weight without flagging or frequently feeling hungry.

THE DIETING EQUATION

Another reason for the rise in obesity is that the simple-minded use of the input/output equation is based on false assumptions. Under some circumstances excess input may be converted to fat; the reverse is not true. Excess fat cannot be shed simply by reducing input. Moreover, if input goes down, output cannot go up, because there is insufficient energy. If the dieting equation were correct, any one of the many special diets around would have solved the fat problem for all time, because no matter what the advertising material says, nearly

WHITE RICE

BELOW *Processed and refined foods lack the vital nutrients required by the body to maintain good health and well-being.*

COOKIES

SPONGE CAKE

LEFT *Everyone has a unique biochemistry. A healthy young man, for example, will have a different metabolism from an overweight fifty-year-old.*

THE FAILURE OF DIETS

The years since 1970 have seen a large number of new specific diets, popularized in magazines and in increasing numbers of books. But as the amount of literature has grown, so too has the number of overweight people.

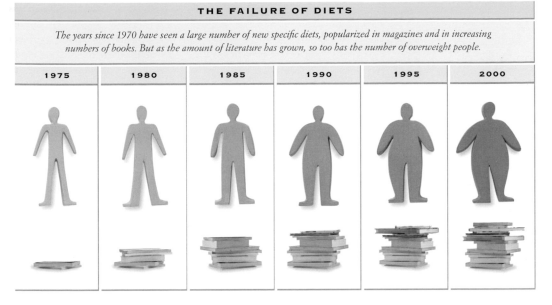

| 1975 | 1980 | 1985 | 1990 | 1995 | 2000 |

every new diet relies on reducing calorie input for it to be effective. (Some hinder nutrient absorption, but this comes to the same thing in the end.) Every diet reduces the amount you eat, even if it denies the fact, by encouraging you to eat as much as you can but limiting your choice. In practical terms it becomes apparent that simply relying on "dieting" can never achieve all that is necessary to lose fat permanently. Further-

more, it seems very likely that any way of eating that causes you to be chronically hungry will tend to make you fat. How can such a thing be true? Television pictures of hungry people in developing countries show clearly that they are not fat. However, it is important to distinguish here between hunger and starvation. People who are starving are losing both fat and lean tissue. Eventually they die since they are either too weak to fight disease-causing

microbes or because the lack of essential nutrients causes a vital part of their system to fail. Feelings of hunger occur when you do not get enough of, or not a full complement of, the correct nutrients that your body requires for its maintenance. People may eat too much on a regular basis but still experience hunger because the types of food they are eating do not contain the right balance of nutrients to balance blood sugar and meet their bodily needs.

ICE CREAM CONSISTS MAINLY OF FAT AND SUGAR

LEFT *The modern Western diet has become far too high in sugar and saturated fat.*

SWEET DRINKS ARE HIGH IN SUGAR

CHIPS CONTAIN FAT AND USUALLY ARTIFICIAL FLAVORINGS

HAMBURGERS CONTAIN SATURATED FATS

FRENCH FRIES ARE HIGH IN FAT

85

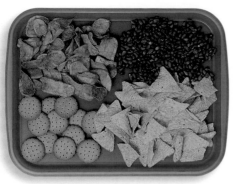

ABOVE *Manufactured snacks leave your body short of essential nutrients.*

HOW CAN HUNGER MAKE YOU FAT?

When you feel the sensation of hunger, whether it is because you are on a diet or due to malnourishment, your body receives the clear message that it is to "prepare for famine". The particular dietary deprivation may be because you are not getting enough minerals and/or vitamins, or you might have an imbalance of carbohydrates, proteins, and fats. If you frequently eat any type of convenience food, it is likely that you have deficiencies and imbalances at all levels.

Whatever your particular "deficiency" or "imbalance" is, your metabolism will register the shortage and the signal it is likely to be sending to your brain is "eat more", making you feel hungry. Therefore, the hunger pangs most dieters have experienced at one time or another may not, in fact, be a signal to consume any food, but may be the body asking for more iron, or zinc, or vitamin B, or protein, to carry out its chemical processes (metabolism) optimally. If your body is unable to maintain a proper metabolic balance because of a deficiency of, say, chromium, your blood sugar swings wildly, causing fat deposition when it rises and hunger as it falls. Moreover, the longer you inflict hunger upon yourself while on a calorie-restricted diet, especially if it involves any kind of "convenience" food, the more your metabolic rate will fall and your body will begin to utilize lean tissue as well as fat. You will lose weight, but most of this will not be fat; you will be losing muscle tissue and materials from vital organs.

FAMINE MESSAGE

To your body, this makes sense. You don't need muscles when you haven't got the energy to use them, and a shutting down of metabolism does not require great cardiac output or efficient detoxification. Since lean muscle tissue has a higher metabolic rate than fat, reducing the former saves on running costs and cuts back on repair bills. Fat will be saved until the last because when your system becomes exhausted, the remaining fat will provide enough energy to keep the vital spark of life burning in the hope that the "famine" will soon end. Also, the more often you go on a "diet" and feel hunger, the quicker your body will respond by conserving fat.

This in turn means that when your weight goes down, your fat goes up; and when your weight starts to come back, fat returns faster than lean tissue. It is thought by some experts that lean tissue loss

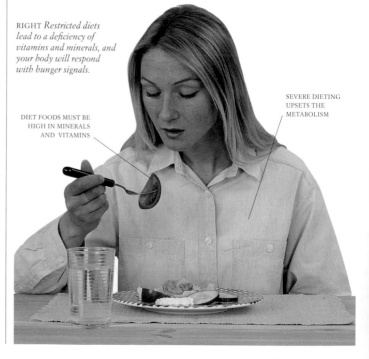

RIGHT *Restricted diets lead to a deficiency of vitamins and minerals, and your body will respond with hunger signals.*

DIET FOODS MUST BE HIGH IN MINERALS AND VITAMINS

SEVERE DIETING UPSETS THE METABOLISM

can take years to be made up, unless you eat in a way that will prevent the "famine" message from getting through and encourage your lean body mass, via sensible exercise and well-balanced dietary protein, to be retained and improved upon.

Because of all the problems with the modern Western diet it comes as no surprise that our bodies are always hungry for the micronutrients that are missing, while at the same time piling on fat from the excesses of refined (micronutrient-stripped) carbohydrates and fats.

Hunger, therefore, can make you fat. Frequent "dieters" will be carrying more fat than would be possible if their diets really worked. Dieters are trying to eat less, yet are getting fatter decade by decade.

Although it may seem that the food industry, the slimming industry, and the media are conspiring to make you fat, there is a way to be naturally slim and healthy.

THINK AND BEHAVE LIKE A SLIM PERSON

The shedding of fat becomes automatic when you start to live in a way that makes fat a disadvantage to your body, and not a survival necessity. The essence of success is to think and behave like a slim person no matter what size you are now. The New Pyramid program helps you do this, and its benefits are listed in the box below.

Successful dieting isn't just trying to find out what works for you if you stick to it, it's about what you can stick to that works! We all know that short-term results are usually fairly easy to achieve, no matter what diet we follow, but how do we make ourselves stick at it? And, if it is an artificial way of eating, should we be thinking of

doing it in the long term anyway? You surely cannot imagine spending the rest of your life drinking very low-calorie milkshakes, and what will be the consequences to your health if you do ?

The best way by far is the New Pyramid program, which will help you to eat more good-quality, nutritional food and restore your hormonal balance. If you feel that supplements are necessary, the most appropriate is a high-potency multivitamin/ multimineral complex, together with essential fatty acids such as fish oils (E.P.A. and D.H.A.) or evening primrose oil.

LEFT *Children are particularly prone to eat junk food, and can get into bad habits at a very young age.*

THE NEW PYRAMID PROGRAM AND DIETING

Although it is intended for all, and not just for slimmers, the New Pyramid program is excellent for all who want to lose weight because it confers many benefits. It will help you:

※ Eat more good-quality food relieved of its chemical load and bursting with micronutrients, antioxidants, and phytochemicals. Eat the correct balance of protein, carbohydrate, and fat; eat when you are hungry and not just for comfort. (Slim people always appear to be truly in tune with their food requirements and naturally stop eating when their bodily requirements are fulfilled).

※ Get your body into hormonal balance so that the controlled burning of your excess fat will maintain you as a naturally slim person.
※ Prevent obsession with food (which itself will cause stress and a slowing of metabolism). Whenever you have to eat out, it is not necessary to decline all the "fattening" foods. Since your basic, everyday eating plan is becoming healthier, you are able to

have the odd "normal" meat without causing too much disruption to your overall fat loss.
※ Use your increasing metabolic capacity to burn fat through increased activity; use exercise to breathe more effectively and increase oxygen levels. (Most slim people are on the go most of the time, are often sporty, and are always enthusiastic and interested in "doing" things).

ESSENTIAL FATS

Despite what we know about fats and their links with excess weight, we must not forget that some fats, the essential fatty acids (E.F.A.s), are indispensable to the body. Nerve cells and brain tissue are insulated (like electric wire) with fat, and the membranes around every cell in our body require fatty acids to control the entry and exit of materials. Enzymes would not be able to work without these membranes. Cholesterol is one of the fats that make up the membranes, and cholesterol is also one of the fats that form the basis for many hormones, including those produced by the adrenal glands and the sex glands. In addition, some fat/protein (lipoprotein) molecules are important as carriers within the blood.

It is quite obvious then that fats are a necessity and that even the leanest tissues require them. However, these fats are mainly those that include a good proportion of the

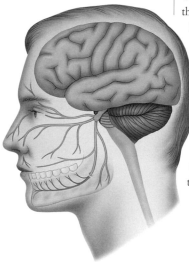

essential fatty acids, and are not based on saturated fat.

Additionally, for those of us living in the temperate zone of the world, there is a need to adapt and cope with a variable climate. This means we are able to put on fat very quickly when food is plentiful and the weather becomes colder. On the other hand, we are designed to lose it only slowly and cautiously as needed or when warmer weather returns. We are conditioned by thousands of years of evolution, and most people who are aware of their bodies will find a little fat going on in the winter and coming off in the spring as part of a natural cycle. If your metabolism is working optimally, this slight amount of winter fat will disappear without effort in the early summer.

SHAPING FAT

In addition to these essential biochemical and structural fats, there is the fat that is found in women, which is specifically associated with the female body shape. We are talking here about true adipose tissue – the fatty layer under the skin. It has distinct extra functions in females, and ignoring these differences can lead to dieting failure no matter how hard you try. This fat gives women their sexually attractive shape and it develops as girls approach maturity. To the adult male this signals that the female is mature and ready to be approached, and to the adult female it is a signal that she

LEFT *Fats are essential – the brain tissue and the nerve cells have a protective outer layer of fat.*

should be treated as a mature female. This fat is of biological necessity for attraction between the sexes and procreation, and is the reason why women have quite a lot more fat then men.

REPRODUCTIVE FAT

Women, during their reproductive years, will have a body that considers a store of fat desirable; this is over and above that required for insulation and body shaping. Biologically, once young females have become shapely and attractive, pregnancy is the next step. Their bodies need to insure that there is a large enough energy store to keep mother and baby well through pregnancy and on into a year or so of breast-feeding. Amenorrhea (lack of menstruation) occurs when female fat falls below a certain level.

So, while women are sexually active, their metabolism encourages extra fat deposition. Although frequent sex and a heightened emotional state can speed up the metabolism, at some point the body may overcompensate once desire is fulfilled, and as sexual exercise decreases, fat may accumulate. On top of this, if your emotional life is stressful, you may turn to food for comfort. Having a good look at how your metabolism is reacting to changing circumstances will enable you to work with your body.

TOXIN STORE

One further function of fat, which has only been briefly mentioned in relation to losing weight, is toxin storage. Many of the substances in our environment are poisonous, and the majority of these are fat-soluble. If your body is unable to metabolize and remove these materials, they tend to become stored away in the fatty tissue. Indeed, the body may even manufacture fat especially for the storage of dangerous substances. Because of the relatively low metabolism of fatty tissue, once toxins are stored here they are likely to remain undisturbed, and the body becomes very reluctant to have them circulate again. The fat becomes persistent. Further fat tends to get dumped in these places because the metabolism has "learned" to do this with a wider range of substances it doesn't like.

LEFT *A woman's rounded shape is both for sexual attractiveness and a sign of preparation for pregnancy.*

If your weight problem is fat retention to protect against toxins, it will become apparent as you lose weight; you will begin to experience some of the symptoms of detoxification, such as a furry tongue, headaches, fever, rash, and tiredness. The only way you will successfully shed fat, especially if you are carrying a lot of it, is by attending to the pollution levels around you and carrying out periodic gentle detoxification regimes (one day a week, a weekend every month, a week every six months, and so on), in between which you can return to a normal eating plan according to the New Pyramid program. Always consult a qualified nutritionist or therapist before beginning any detoxification program.

HOW DRUGS CAUSE WEIGHT GAIN

Some drugs may make it harder for you to lose weight, either because of a tendency to encourage fluid retention, or by interfering with metabolism. Despite this, a period of detoxification, a change to a nutrient-dense diet, and a moderate increase in exercise will still enable you to lose weight.

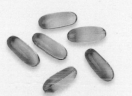

ABOVE *Tell your physician if you are taking supplements in addition to prescribed drugs.*

The prescription drugs that can have weight gain as a direct effect are:
❋ hormones such as oral contraceptives, hormone replacement therapies, and male sex hormones
❋ drugs for diabetes
❋ drugs acting on the central nervous system, such as antidepressants, and tranquilizers.
❋ drugs for prevention of migraine
❋ drugs for heart disease and high blood pressure
❋ anti-inflammatory drugs
❋ antihistamines

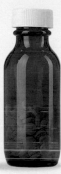

LEFT *Prescription drugs can have an adverse effect on the metabolism.*

FLUCTUATIONS IN WOMEN'S APPETITES

If you are female and find that even on the New Pyramid diet you have times of the month when your appetite increases and you go out of control, this section is just for you. It applies to women who are currently experiencing a regular menstrual cycle (whatever the length). It is not suitable for individuals who have had their ovaries or uterus removed, for anyone suffering absence of periods (for whatever reason), for postmenopausal women (though some may benefit), or for those on H.R.T. or steroid hormones.

How many times have you heard, or you may even experience this yourself, that for two or three weeks of each month a woman is a normal confident person who finds it relatively easy to stick to a good healthy diet in her battle to lose weight? However, a week or ten days before her period is due she begins to feel fat and ugly and eats everything in sight. Because she gets depressed, grumpy, and very tired, and begins to believe she is fat and ugly, her diet goes out of the window. She may feel bloated and feel she wants to pick constantly at chocolate, bread, and cookies.

There seems to be a very fine dividing line between true P.M.S. and how a woman normally feels as her menstrual cycle unfolds, but in any case, these monthly appetite swings can ruin even the best diet, especially since it is during the increased-appetite phase that we feel less inclined to exercise. As we approach menopause, we may find that we exchange symptoms of P.M.S. for those of "the change", but even in many postmenopausal women, a regular cycle of mood swings and appetite changes still seems to occur.

UNDERSTANDING THE FEMALE CYCLE

The female hormone cycle consists of five stages (left). Most of the problems associated with periods occur during stage four and intensify in stage five when both estrogen and progesterone are very low. This time of the month is often connected, even in the healthiest of women, with mood changes, tearfulness, and irritability. It is also the time when appetite increases along, obviously, with food intake.

Scientific research has found that although a woman's daytime resting

THE FEMALE HORMONE CYCLE

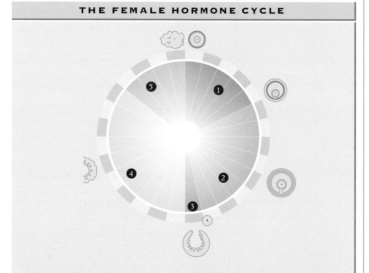

Stage One
Menstruation, lasting about four days (and sometimes as long as ten days). The first day of bleeding is day one.

Stage Two
The Follicular Phase (so called because it is within this time that hormones from the pituitary stimulate the ripening of egg follicles on the surface of the ovaries). This includes the days of bleeding and lasts up to the point of ovulation.

Stage Three
Ovulation, in response to a sudden surge of estrogen, occurs around day 14 of the cycle, when an egg is released from the ovary.

Stage Four
The Luteal Phase (the empty follicle becomes a gland called the corpus luteum). Secretion of estrogen and more importantly progesterone (the pregnancy hormone) occurs to prepare the womb lining for receiving a fertilized ovum, should conception occur; this lasts from day 15 to day 28.

Stage Five
The Premenstrual Phase usually lasts from around day 24 to day 28. The levels of estrogen and progesterone suddenly plummet to very low levels (in response to the absence of a fertilized egg).

metabolic rate does not change much throughout her cycle, nevertheless at night it is increased in the ten nights before each period by up to 10 percent. This means your body burns off calories more efficiently in the second half of the cycle.

CYCLICAL EATING

It has been apparent for some time now that bodily changes occur in a rhythmic way throughout the day, month, and season. The controlling mechanism occurs at the base of the brain in the hypothalamus. This part of the brain is very near to both the pituitary gland, which is the master endocrine gland orchestrating all of the other endocrine glands in their hormonal secretion and regulatory processes, not least of which is that of menstruation, and the centers controlling appetite and sleep.

The body-rhythm center in the hypothalamus releases chemical messengers in timed sequences that affect other centers in the hypothalamus and pituitary gland, resulting in a series of processes that are switched off and on depending on the unique biological rhythm or "biorhythms" of the body. These relate to the thousands of fluctuations in body chemistry that occur naturally, not only in humans but also in animals and plants, each day, month, and year of existence.

RIGHT *Most of the problems associated with periods come together at the end of the menstrual cycle.*

For a woman, the most important rhythm related to appetite and weight is the menstrual cycle. Metabolic rate, particularly at night, is elevated from around day 15 to the end of the menstrual cycle. Cyclical eating attempts to finetune these biorhythmic changes into three stages related to the variability of the woman's energy requirement.

During the first 14 days of your cycle (starting with day one when you start bleeding) you can restrict your eating, since your appetite will be lower. During the phase from day 15 to day 23 you may increase the amount of food you eat. More complex carbohydrate can be eaten, appropriately balanced with protein, or you could increase the number of healthy snacks, such as seeds, fruits and nuts.

During the phase from day 24 to 28, when appetite has really increased, you can indulge even more according to your appetite.

HOW ARE YOU AFFECTED BY YOUR HORMONAL CYCLE?

Give simple "yes" or "no" answers to the following questions.

● Are there certain times of the month when dieting is a real struggle for you, or you may give up altogether?
● Do you find yourself craving chocolate, stodgy foods, carbohydrate, or sweet things a few days before a period is due?
● Do you become depressed and think that you will never be slim?
● Are you fed up with your weight constantly going up and down?
● Has there been any reduction in normal sexual interest?
● Do you suffer from emotional swings, tearfulness, etc. in a regular cycle?
● Do your breasts become tender at the same time each month?
● Does your skin change to become drier or greasier in a regular cycle?
● Does your energy level drop considerably just before a period is due?
● Does your appetite increase just before a period?

SCORING

If you have said "yes" to one or two only of the above, then your system would appear to be only mildly affected by hormonal cycles. If, however, you have said "yes" to all, or nearly all of these questions, it may be that you have P.M.S. and are quite strongly affected by your hormonal cycles, so much so that a cyclical diet would suit you.

Self-help for Common Ailments

THE FOLLOWING *pages contain a general guide to self-help for many common diseases. Where lists of "Suggested Supplements" are quoted, it is not intended that all the supplements be used at the same time, simply that these preparations that have been found helpful. Never self-prescribe herbs, amino acids, or non-standard/single nutritional accessories; obtain the help of a nutritional therapist.*

LEFT *The herb* Aloe vera *has a soothing effect on the gut and is used to treat skin problems.*

NUTRITIONAL ACCESSORY SUPPLEMENTS

NUTRITIONAL ACCESSORY	HELPFUL FOR	NUTRITIONAL ACCESSORY	HELPFUL FOR
N-acetyl glucosamine	Poor integrity of intestinal mucous membranes	**Glycosamino-glycans**	Atherosclerosis/thrombosis
Anthocyanidins	Inflammation and oxidation/high uric acid levels/capillary fragility/poor eyesight	**Grapefruit seed extract**	Parasitic/fungal infections of the gut
		Green-lipped mussel	Osteoarthritic pain and stiffness
		Hesperidin	Poor collagen integrity/poor gut lining/capillary fragility/menopausal problems
Antioxidants	Inflammation and oxidation		
Beet extract	Toxicity/poor blood function	**Hydrochloric acid (betaine hydrochloride)**	Gastric infections/poor mineral absorption/allergy
Bioflavonoids	Circulatory problems/capillary fragility/poor healing and repair of tissue/poor collagen maintenance		
		Lactobacillus acidophilus	Poor gut flora/candida overgrowth
Bromelain	Poor protein digestion/food sensitivity		
Butyric acid	Dysbiosis/irritated gut lining	**Lecithin**	Poor fat metabolism/nerve problems
Cabagin	Peptic ulcers/dysbiosis	**Lipoic acid**	Cataracts/glaucoma/diabetes
Caprylic acid	*Candida albicans* infestations	**Licorice root**	Ulcerated gut lining
Cellulose	Constipation	**Manuka honey**	Indigestion/peptic ulcers
Charcoal (activated)	Flatulence/poor fatty acid levels in gut	**S-methylmethionine**	Intestinal irritation/dysbiosis
Chondroitin sulfate	Poor cartilage formation/joint problems	**Octacosanol (wheatgerm oil)**	Poor nerve insulation
Cranberry	Cystitis	**Pectin**	Constipation/high cholesterol
Digestive enzymes (lipase, amylase, protease)	Poor digestion	**Peppermint oil**	Bowel irritation/flatulence
		Phosphatidyl serine	Poor memory
		Propolis	Poor immune function
Evening primrose oil	Inflammation/hormonal problems	**Rooibosh tea**	Intestinal irritation
Fish oils (D.H.A. and E.P.A.)	Inflammation/poor circulation/heart problems	**Spirulina (algae)**	Poor nutrient levels (especially amino acids)
Fructo-oligosaccharides	Poor gut flora/low levels of *Bifido* bacteria	**Starflower (borage)**	General inflammation/hormonal problems
Gamma-oryzanol	Poor stomach muscle tone/gastritis	**Tea-tree oil (external)**	Skin infections/ringworm/pulled muscles
		Tocotrienol	High cholesterol
		Wild yam	Female hormone imbalance/menopause

AMINO ACIDS USED IN NUTRITIONAL HEALING

NUTRITIONAL ACCESSORY	HELPFUL FOR	NUTRITIONAL ACCESSORY	HELPFUL FOR
L-alanine	Prostate problems	L-glutamine	Intestinal lining problems/poor
L-arginine	Poor sperm production		thyroid function/alcoholism/
Aspartic acid	Imbalance of cellular minerals/		poor muscle tone
	low energy	L-glutathione	Detoxification
L-carnitine	Heart and circulatory problems	L-glycine	Prostate problems/detoxification
L-cysteine	Poor detoxification and absorption,	L-lysine	Cold sores/shingles/genital herpes
	especially vitamin B6/poor hair growth	L-methionine	Poor detoxification of protein
L-cystine	Heavy metal toxicity/poor healing		by-products/nerve problems
	after trauma	DL-phenylalanine	Generalized pain
Glutamic acid	Prostate problems	Taurine	Gallstones/hyperactivity/poor
			brain function

BOTANICALS USED IN NUTRITIONAL HEALING

NUTRITIONAL ACCESSORY	HELPFUL FOR	NUTRITIONAL ACCESSORY	HELPFUL FOR
Agnus castus	Premenstrual/menstrual problems	Ginseng (Siberian)	Stress/impotence
Alfalfa	Fluid retention/colon problems	Golden seal	Constipation/toxic liver
Aloe vera	Inflammation/skin problems/	Gota kola	Poor memory/high blood pressure
	burns/arthritis	Grapefruit seed	
Astragalus	Poor immune function/	extract	Gut parasites
	interferon insufficiency	Hawthorn	Stress/high cholesterol/diarrhea
Bilberry	Menstrual cramps/poor collagen	Hops	Insomnia/high uric acid & fluid levels
	formation	Kelp	Low iodine levels/low thyroid
Berberis	Dysbiosis/gut spasms/poor immune		function
	function/poor liver function	Licorice	Stomach and intestinal irritation/
Boswellia	Muscle and joint pain/stiffness		poor mucus production
Cat's claw	Poor immune function	Marshmallow	Epithelial irritation
Celery seed	Excess acid/fluid retention/arthritis/	Motherwort	Menstrual and menopausal problems
	high blood pressure	Passion flower	Stress/insomnia
Cinnamon	Intestinal cramps	Pau d'arco	Fungal infections in intestinal tract
Clove oil	Spasm of intestinal tract	Pygeum africanum	Prostate problems
Cranberry	Bladder and urethral infections	Psyllium	Constipation/toxicity of colon
Dandelion	Poor hepatic balance/poor bile	Rhubarb	Low levels of phytoesterols
	production/blood problems	Rutin	Eye problems/capillary fragility
Devil's claw	Arthritic pain and stiffness	Sanguinaria	Bronchial & periodontal infections
Echinacea	Poor immune function/flatulence	Saw palmetto	Prostate problems
Elderberry extract	Poor immune function/influenza	Silymarin	Toxic liver/alcohol misuse/
Feverfew	Headaches/migraine	(Milk thistle)	poor hepatic balance
Garlic	Poor immune function/circulatory	Slippery elm	Toxic and irritated intestinal tract
	problems/high cholesterol	St. John's wort	Depression and anxiety
Ginger	Nausea/hot flashes/menstrual pain	Valerian	Stress/insomnia/intestinal irritation
Ginkgo biloba	Poor circulation/tinnitus/asthma	White willow	Pain/inflammation/stomach irritation

Disorders of the Heart, Circulation, and Blood

THE CIRCULATORY SYSTEM *is an amazing and complicated network consisting of a pump (the heart) and its connecting tubes (arteries, arterioles, capillaries, venules, and veins). Over the course of an average lifetime, the heart will pump 55 million gallons of blood through 60,000 miles of blood vessels. The whole purpose of this system is to deliver supplies of oxygen, nutrients, and other substances to the body's 60 trillion cells, and to remove carbon dioxide and wastes.*

CAUSES OF CARDIOVASCULAR DISEASE

Most diseases of the cardiovascular system stem from a too high intake of saturated and hydrogenated fats, which attach to the walls of blood vessels and form atheromatous plaques, constricting the flow of blood. A dietary excess of sugar and refined carbohydrates can also create plaques, because of the conversion of excess sugar to fat. High levels of some refined carbohydrates also raise blood triglyceride levels and increase platelet adhesiveness. Additionally, the clotting time of the blood may be reduced, leading to a higher risk of blood clots forming and blocking blood vessels completely. Lack of essential fatty acids can lead to "stiffened" red blood cells, which are unable to squeeze through the fine capillaries, this may lead to chronic fatigue. Diets high in salt can cause fluid retention and other problems that lead to high blood pressure (hypertension). Increased capillary fragility occurs when diets are high in refined and processed food, a condi-

---

HEART DISEASE AND CIRCULATORY DISORDERS

Nutritional considerations
+ excess saturated fats
+ excess use of hydrogenated, overheated, or oxidized vegetable oils
+ trans-fatty acids
+ excess refined carbohydrates and sugars
+ high intake of foods fortified with vitamin D (vitamin D excess)
+ excess dairy products
+ vitamin and mineral deficiencies
+ excess coffee and alcohol
+ high homocysteine levels
+ overweight

Maximize
+ Foods such as dark green and orange vegetables, peas, oats, onions, garlic, fresh wheatgerm, mixed seeds, spouted seeds, lecithin granules.
Eat
+ Mainly vegetable protein. Eat oily fish two or three times a week.
Avoid
+ Salt, coffee, sugar, refined grains, hydrogenated fats and trans-fats, fried foods, fatty or processed meats, full-fat milk and cheese, cream. Minimize intake of alcohol (two units once or twice a week).

SUGGESTED SUPPLEMENTS

A multivitamin/multimineral containing vitamin A, vitamin B-complex (especially B₆) with folic acid, vitamin C, bioflavonoids especially quercetin, vitamin E (only 100iu per day if on blood-thinning drugs), magnesium, selenium, chromium, and copper; a high-potency garlic supplement; Ginkgo biloba; Aloe vera; L-carnitine, fish oils, linseed (flax seed) oil, and lecithin

---

tion exacerbated by smoking, excess alcohol, and lack of exercise.

The red blood cells need various nutrients to keep them working properly, including essential fatty acids, several vitamins (especially the B vitamins), and minerals especially iron. If any of these nutrients are low, anemia and other blood diseases can develop.

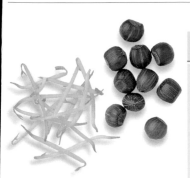

ABOVE *Beansprouts help lower blood pressure, while nuts can help combat anemia.*

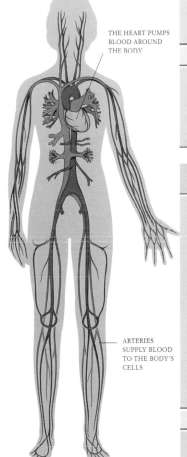

THE HEART PUMPS BLOOD AROUND THE BODY

ARTERIES SUPPLY BLOOD TO THE BODY'S CELLS

ABOVE *The main circulatory system of the blood.*

HIGH BLOOD PRESSURE

Nutritional considerations
✛ excess salt, sugar, tea, and coffee
✛ saturated fats, hydrogenated fats, and trans-fatty acids
✛ excess alcohol
✛ poor calcium/magnesium balance
✛ low fiber intake
✛ obesity

Maximize
✛ Foods containing pectins, such as apples and carrots, and eat a large proportion of potassium-rich foods. (See macrominerals, page 37).

Eat
✛ A basically vegetarian diet for three to six months; include a little oily fish twice a week and live yogurt daily. Eat alfalfa spouts and other sprouted seeds and beans. Add ground linseeds (flax seeds) to your seed mixture of sunflower, pumpkin, and sesame.

Avoid
✛ Salt, coffee, alcohol, sugar, refined grains, hydrogenated fats and trans-fats, fried foods, meat, full-fat milk and cheese, cream. Avoid grapefruit juice if on calcium channel blockers.

SUGGESTED SUPPLEMENTS

Vitamin C with bioflavonoids (or anthocyanidins, such as grape seed, bilberry, and pine bark), or a high-potency antioxidant including betacarotene, vitamin C, vitamin E, and selenium; vitamin B6; magnesium; fish oils or edible linseed (flax) oil; garlic; lecithin; Aloe vera; palm oil or rice bran tocotrienols.

ANEMIA

Nutritional considerations
✛ insufficiency of iron, vitamins B6, B12, C, E, and folic acid
✛ zinc-induced copper deficiency
✛ excess onion/garlic/root ginger
✛ excess alcohol

Maximize
✛ Mineral- and vitamin-rich liver and other organ meats once or twice a week (but not if you are pregnant or are planning a pregnancy), make sure you eat plenty of fish and/or vegetable proteins (pulses [legumes], nuts, and seeds).

Eat
✛ Plenty of green leafy vegetables and dried fruit such as apricots and figs, and molasses. Increase amount of freshly ground mixed seeds, especially linseed (flax seed), and wheatgerm.

Avoid
✛ Foods and drinks that inhibit iron absorption, such as coffee, tea, alcohol, and wheat bran. Avoid processes that cause loss of vitamins B and C, such as incorrect storage, long cooking times, and consumption of diuretics. Reduce onions and garlic.

SUGGESTED SUPPLEMENTS

Multivitamin/multimineral with a good supply of all B vitamins, but not including iron (iron inhibits absorption of other nutrients), plus a separate iron supplement taken, in chelated form, at a different meal; vitamin C; Aloe vera.

Disorders of the Immune System

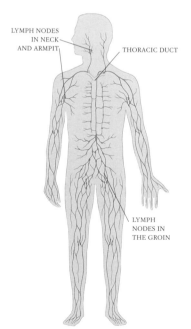

RIGHT
Garlic has been used for centuries as an aid to disease resistance.

THE IMMUNE SYSTEM *is the part of our body that protects us against infectious disease and tissues that grow to become non-self tissues (such as cancers and tumors). There are many different types of micro-organisms (prions, viruses, bacteria, yeasts, molds) that have the power to harm us.*

The body has two lines of defense. Firstly, micro-organisms can be prevented from entering the body; for this we need a healthy covering of skin, normal acid levels in the stomach, and ciliated cells and mucus lining the airways to trap and inactivate any microbes. The second line of defense is to disarm those that inevitably do enter using various white cells, which engulf microbes, release antibodies, or release substances to kill or neutralize them.

LYMPH NODES
IN NECK
AND ARMPIT

THORACIC DUCT

LYMPH
NODES IN
THE GROIN

**THE LYMPHATHIC SYSTEM;
INVOLVED IN IMMUNITY**

A.I.D.S AND H.I.V

Nutritional considerations
✹ low intake of antioxidant nutrients
✹ low intake of E.F.A.s (essential fatty acids)
✹ generalized vitamin (especially B$_1$ and C) and mineral deficiencies
✹ dysbiosis of gut (especially overgrowth of molds and yeasts) – may need a detoxification diet
✹ food allergy/intolerance – may need a hypoallergenic diet
✹ acidosis
✹ refined carbohydrates and sugar
✹ dairy products
Maximize
✹ Intake of antioxidant vegetables and fruit, especially dark green and orange vegetables and fruit, shiitake mushrooms, and garlic.
Eat
✹ Raw vegetables, sprouted seeds, and pulses (legumes) daily, plenty of freshly ground mixed seeds (especially pumpkin), and oily fish.
Avoid
✹ Refined carbohydrate, sugar.

SUPPLEMENTS

Antioxidant formula; vitamin A; high levels of vitamin C; high-potency vitamin B-complex, with good levels of B$_1$; evening primrose oil and fish oils or linseed (flax seed) oil.

CHRONIC FATIGUE SYNDROME

Nutritional considerations
✹ food allergy/intolerance – may need a hypoallergenic diet, and/or food combining diet
✹ poor level of nutrients (poor digestion and absorption)
✹ poor immune function (overgrowth of *Candida,* etc.)
✹ poor intake of E.F.A.s (essential fatty acids)
Maximize
✹ Intake of lightly steamed vegetables and freshly ground mixed seeds, as well as antioxidant nutrients.
Eat
✹ Tofu, millet, quinoa, "seed" vegetables e.g. green beans, seeds and some nuts, and fish.
Avoid
✹ All stimulants (tea, coffee, alcohol, colas), "rich" foods, common allergenic foods, additives and refined food, and sugar. Minimize foods that are hard to digest (e.g. red meat and dairy products).

SUPPLEMENTS

High-quality multivitamin/ multimineral; maximum vitamin B$_{12}$, vitamin C, magnesium and zinc; antioxidants; fish oils or linseed oil; evening primrose oil; Echinacea.

POOR DISEASE RESISTANCE AND WOUND HEALING

Nutritional considerations
❀ low levels of vitamin C, bioflavonoids, antioxidants, and zinc
❀ excess toxins in food and water
❀ excess refined carbohydrate; excess carbohydrate generally (especially sweet foods)
❀ excess animal proteins, especially those from dairy food
❀ excess alcohol
Maximize
❀ Vegetables and fruit high in vitamins A and C, freshly ground mixed seeds (especially pumpkin), garlic, and onions.
Eat
❀ Organic products. Drink elderberry cordial (especially for influenza).
Avoid
❀ Alcohol, candy, tea, coffee, milk, and cheese. Minimize grain carbohydrate (but not carbohydrate from vegetables).

SUPPLEMENTS

Vitamins A and C, and maximum levels of zinc; vitamin B-complex; high-potency garlic; propolis; Echinacea herb; Astralagus herb; Aloe vera; elderberry extract.

TUMORS AND CANCER

Nutritional considerations
❀ lack of nutrient-dense food
❀ saturated, hydrogenated fats, and trans-fatty acids
❀ low dietary fiber
❀ excess refined food and sugar
❀ excess alcohol
❀ excess smoked, pickled, and salt-cured food
❀ "soft" water (hard water protects against digestive cancers)
❀ chlorinated water (may be related to bladder cancer)
❀ polluted food and water
Maximize
❀ Intake of antioxidant nutrients, raw and lightly cooked vegetables, and freshly ground seeds.
Eat
❀ Tomatoes, broccoli, Brussels sprouts, hot peppers, onions, apples, pink grapefruit, watermelon, guava, raspberries, strawberries, wheatgrass, shiitake mushrooms, soy, and beans.
Avoid
❀ Saturated fats, processed fat/oils, refined food, stimulants.

SUPPLEMENTS

Anthocyanidins; natural beta-carotene; vitamins B6, folic acid, C and E; magnesium; selenium; zinc, coenzyme Q10; Lactobacillus acidophilus; Omega-3 oils; butyric acid; garlic; Aloe vera.

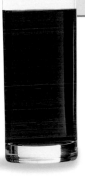

LEFT AND BELOW *Cranberry juice can boost the immune system. Fresh green vegetables can protect the body against cancers and tumors.*

COLD SORES, GENITAL HERPES AND SHINGLES

Nutritional considerations
❀ arginine-rich foods (wheat, almonds, peanuts, bacon, chicken)
❀ citrus and acid diet
❀ low vitamin levels
Maximize
❀ Vegetables and fruit high in vitamins A and C
Eat
❀ Garlic and onion.
Avoid
❀ Alcohol, candy, tea, coffee, and arginine-rich foods.

SUPPLEMENTS

Lysine (appears to inhibit replication of the virus); vitamins A and C, selenium, and other antioxidants; Echinacea herb; Aloe vera.

CANDIDIASIS AND THRUSH

Nutritional considerations
❀ excess refined carbohydrate and sweet foods
❀ foods containing yeast
❀ deficiency of vitamin B-complex
Maximize
❀ Vegetables and fruit high in vitamins A and C, and antioxidants.
Eat
❀ Garlic, olive oil, raw vegetables, and oily fish.

SUPPLEMENTS

Vitamins A, B-complex; additional B6; vitamin C; vitamin E; zinc; high-potency garlic; Lactobacillus acidophilus; grapefruit seed extract; Aloe vera; magnesium.

Disorders of the Nervous System

ABOVE *A* Ginkgo biloba *supplement may help sufferers from Alzheimer's.*

THE CENTRAL NERVOUS *system comprises the brain and spinal cord. It is intricately connected to the peripheral nervous system, which comprises all the nerve fibers (neurones) throughout the body. Electrical stimuli are received, converted into an electrical message and sent via sensory neurones to the brain. The autonomic nervous system involves electrical signals between the brain and the organs. Voluntary actions occur when the brain sends electrical messages to our muscles.*

Electrical messages occur because of the activities of the minerals sodium, potassium, calcium, and magnesium. Pollutants, such as drugs and heavy metals, can interfere with electrical pathways.

For the nervous system to work correctly many different substances are required. If too much or too little neurotransmitter is produced, this may lead to depression. If the body has low levels of the minerals involved in transmission, e.g., sodium, potassium, calcium, and magnesium, then nerve tissue cannot work effectively. The "insulation" around nerves, called the myelin sheath, is made up of very specific types of fatty acids. Reduction of this insulation layer causes nerves to misfire or to fail in transmitting the impulse to its destination. These effects can be seen in diseases such as multiple sclerosis.

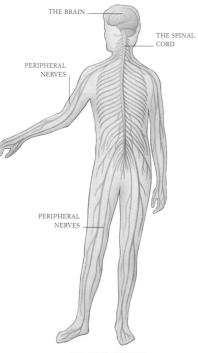

THE BRAIN

THE SPINAL CORD

PERIPHERAL NERVES

PERIPHERAL NERVES

THE NERVOUS SYSTEM

DEPRESSION AND PROBLEMS OF THE MIND

Nutritional considerations
+ additives, coloring, sweeteners
+ excess white sugar
+ excess refined and processed food
+ foods high in tyramine (e.g. cheese and red wine)
+ caffeine
+ generalized mineral and vitamin deficiencies – may need a food combining diet
+ essential fatty acid deficiency
+ alcohol and drugs
+ food allergy/intolerance – may need a hypoallergenic diet

+ heavy metal toxicity in food, water, and air (e.g. lead, cadmium, mercury) – may need a detoxification diet

Maximize
+ Intake of raw and lightly cooked vegetables and fish, and ground mixed seeds, including linseeds.

Eat
+ Organic produce whenever possible. Eat fresh and dried fruit as sources of sugar.

Avoid
+ Refined foods, additives, sugar, alcohol, tea, coffee, colas, and cheese.

SUGGESTED SUPPLEMENTS

A good-quality multivitamin/multimineral (containing maximum levels of vitamin B-complex and folic acid, vitamin C, calcium, magnesium, and zinc); vitamin C to total maximum level; lecithin; L-carnitine; DL-phenylalanine; phosphatidyl serine; evening primrose oil; Ginkgo biloba; methionine (to detox the liver). Additionally, for helping with depression, St. John's wort herb.

ALZHEIMER'S DISEASE AND DEMENTIA

Nutritional considerations
✣ low-serum vitamin B (especially B12) levels
✣ excess refined and processed food
✣ low intake of vegetables, fruit, and wholegrains
✣ excess saturated fat/low essential fatty acids
✣ poor nutrient absorption
✣ food allergy/intolerance – may need a hypoallergenic diet
✣ aluminum toxicity (from the environment, especially cooking utensils) – may need detoxification
Maximize
✣ Intake of raw or lightly cooked vegetables and fruit, antioxidant-rich vegetables and fruit (especially garlic), seeds, seed oils, and nuts.
Eat
✣ Fermented foods (yogurt, miso, tempeh); sip cider vinegar with at least one meal. Take wheatgerm or oatgerm, and molasses daily.
Avoid
✣ Refined, processed, overcooked foods and alcohol.

SUPPLEMENTS

Multivitamin/multimineral with maximum levels of B vitamins, calcium, magnesium, zinc, silica; antioxidants; Ginkgo biloba; phosphatidyl choline (lecithin); phosphatidyl serine.

BELOW AND RIGHT *Too much refined food and fat can lead to Alzheimer's. Maximize your intake of seed oils and wholegrains.*

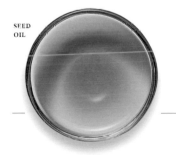

SEED OIL

MULTIPLE SCLEROSIS

Nutritional considerations
✣ excess saturated fat/low intake of essential fatty acids
✣ excessive meat and dairy foods
✣ gluten-containing grains
✣ yeast
✣ low intake of antioxidants
Maximize
✣ Intake of raw and lightly cooked vegetables, mixed seeds, and antioxidant-containing vegetables.
Eat
✣ Gluten-free grains, sprouted seeds, and live yogurt.

SUPPLEMENTS

Multivitamin/multimineral with good levels of vitamin B complex, and vitamin C, calcium, magnesium, selenium, and zinc; fish oils or linseed (flax seed) oil; Aloe vera.

PARKINSON'S DISEASE

Nutritional considerations
✣ amino acid imbalance
✣ low levels of certain vitamins
✣ manganese and heavy metal toxicity
Maximize
✣ Intake of fruit, vegetables and wholegrain carbohydrates (exclude wheat), seed oils, olive oil and nuts.
Eat
✣ Organic produce.
Avoid
✣ Refined, processed, high protein foods, aluminum cooking pots.

SUPPLEMENTS

Multivitamin/multimineral with good levels of calcium, magnesium and silica; vitamin B-complex, C, E; selenium; iron; wheatgerm oil.

STRESS, INSOMNIA, AND GENERALIZED PAIN

Nutritional considerations
✣ excess refined and processed foods
✣ food additives/preservatives
✣ low intake of magnesium and calcium
✣ vitamin B-complex deficiency
✣ low intake of antioxidant-containing foods
✣ overeating
✣ excess caffeine and alcohol
✣ excess sodium (salt) and iodine
✣ food allergy/intolerance –
✣ toxic heavy metals in food, water, air (e.g. lead, cadmium) – may need a detoxification diet
Maximize
✣ Intake of antioxidant-containing fruit and vegetables, raw and dark green vegetables, ground mixed seeds (sesame).
Eat
✣ Wheatgerm or oatgerm and live yogurt daily.
Avoid
✣ Refined, processed foods, caffeine, additives, alcohol, salt.

SUPPLEMENTS

Vitamin B complex, vitamin C; antioxidants; lecithin; calcium-magnesium formula; Siberian ginseng herbal combinations (e.g. valerian/passionflower); camomile; fish oils; DL-phenylalanine.

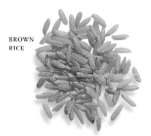

BROWN RICE

Disorders of the Skeletal System

THE SKELETAL SYSTEM *is made up of 206 bones. Joints, held together by ligaments, enable the bones to articulate with each other. Muscles are attached to bones by tendons, and cartilage insures they work smoothly. All of these tissues are made up of proteins such as collagen and elastin, and a host of different minerals (calcium, magnesium, phosphorus, fluoride, and boron).*

ABOVE *Antioxidant fruit such as grapes helps skeletal disorders.*

Calcium and other minerals are also required by the blood and body tissues for efficient metabolism. When calcium is low in these tissues, then the body will extract the calcium it needs from the bones. Conversely, when calcium is in excess (either because of a simple excess or because of insufficient magnesium), it may be deposited in inappropriate places, such as plaques in arteries, lumps and bumps in joints, and in soft tissue such as muscle and liver.

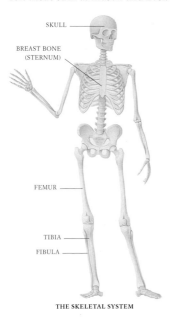

SKULL

BREAST BONE (STERNUM)

FEMUR

TIBIA

FIBULA

THE SKELETAL SYSTEM

ARTHRITIS AND FIBROMYALGIA

Nutritional considerations
+ red meat and staturated fats
+ dairy foods high in lactic acid
+ nightshade foods (potatoes etc.)
+ excessive intake of calcium and sodium (salt)
+ excess refined carbohydrates
+ insufficient raw vegetables
+ stimulants (tea, coffee etc.)
+ acid fruit
+ excess weight

Maximize
+ Intake of antioxidant vegetables and fruit, bioflavonoids, mixed seeds, lightly cooked vegetables.

Eat
+ A mainly vegetarian diet with a little oily fish two or three times a week. Eat Jerusalem artichokes. Drink vegetable juice (e.g. carrot) instead of fruit juice.

Avoid
+ Red meat, dairy foods, saturated fat, salty or pickled foods, additives, acid fruit, nightshade foods, tea, coffee and sugar drinks.

SUPPLEMENTS

Vitamin B-complex; vitamins C and E; high-potency antioxidants; fish oils; glucosamine sulphate; green-lipped mussel extract.

OSTEOPOROSIS

Nutritional considerations
+ excess protein, fat, dairy food
+ poor levels of vitamins C, D, magnesium, boron
+ poor calcium absorption
+ poor levels of gut bacteria
+ excess candy, salt, and refined carbohydrates
+ stomach acid deficiency
+ excess alcohol and coffee

Maximize
+ Intake of vegetables and fruit, ground mixed seeds (especially sesame and pumpkin).

Eat
+ Raw vegetables, sprouted seeds, pulses (legumes), live yogurt. Eat fish, soy, and nuts three times a week. Drink a little cider vinegar with one meal a day.

Avoid
+ Nightshade foods (tomato, potato, eggplant, sweet peppers), refined carbohydrate and sweet foods, cereals, animal proteins (except fish and yogurt), coffee, alcohol, fluoride toothpastes.

SUPPLEMENTS

Multivitamin/multimineral with vitamin B-complex, C, E, zinc, copper, iron, calcium/magnesium, boron silica, and molybdenum.

LOW BACK PAIN AND SCIATICA

Nutritional considerations
✛ obesity
✛ protein and/or calcium deficiency (caused by poor intake or poor absorption)
✛ poor level of stomach acid – may need a food-combining diet
✛ insufficient intake of dark green vegetables
✛ low intake of vitamin C
✛ excess refined carbohydrates
Maximize
✛ Intake of dark green vegetables, and vegetables and fruit containing vitamin C.
Eat
✛ Plant proteins (soy, pulses [legumes], seed vegetables), and a little oily fish.
✛ Drink a little diluted freshly squeezed lemon juice or cider vinegar with main meal of day.
Avoid
✛ Intake of dairy foods and red meat, alcohol, refined carbohydrates, and sugar.

SUPPLEMENTS

High-potency vitamin B-complex; vitamin C and bioflavonoids; balanced calcium/magnesium complex with boron; bromelain; digestive enzymes; DL-phenylalanine (as painkiller).

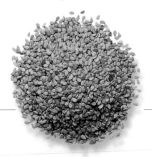

BELOW *Ground mixed seeds, such as sesame, can help many conditions.*

GOUT

Nutritional considerations
✛ excess meat, carbohydrates
✛ excess alcohol and coffee
✛ excess purine-containing foods (organ meats, shellfish, oats, yeast)
Maximize
✛ Antioxidant vegetables and fruit.
Eat
✛ Low acid-forming grains (millet, corn, buckwheat), deep-sea white fish, free-range eggs, low-fat cheese, goat's milk and yogurt.
Avoid
✛ Refined carbohydrates, offal.

SUPPLEMENTS

High-potency antioxidants with maximum levels of vitamins A, C, and E, bioflavonoids; vitamin B-complex; lecithin; bromelain; linseed (flax seed) oil; Aloe vera

CARPAL TUNNEL SYNDROME

Nutritional considerations
✛ low levels of B vitamins
✛ excess refined carbohydrates
✛ excess vitamin D/calcium
✛ excess alcohol and other stimulants
Maximize
✛ Antioxidant fruit and vegetables and ground mixed seeds.
Eat
✛ Extra molasses daily, and add wheatgerm or oatgerm to food.

SUPPLEMENTS

A high-potency vitamin B-complex; calcium and magnesium balanced formula (2:1 magnesium to calcium); fish oils or linseed (flax seed) oil.

TENDONITIS

Nutritional considerations
✛ toxic system
✛ food allergy/intolerance
✛ foods fortified with vitamin D
✛ excess calcium
Maximize
✛ Intake of fresh antioxidant vegetables and fruit and freshly ground mixed seeds.
Eat
✛ Vegetable and brown rice diet for a few days to remove toxicity.
Avoid
✛ Dairy foods (minimize meat).

SUPPLEMENTS

Vitamin C; vitamin E; betacarotene; Aloe vera

SPRAINS

Nutritional considerations
✛ low levels of vitamin C
✛ low levels of antioxidants
✛ excess calcium
Maximize
✛ Antioxidant nutrients, mixed seeds (especially sesame and pumpkin).
Eat
✛ Vegetables and fruit, expecially those rich in vitamin C.
Avoid
✛ Meat, dairy food, alcohol, and coffee.

SUPPLEMENTS

High-potency antioxidants; maximum vitamin C; silica; glucosamine (N-acetyl glucosamine); Aloe vera.

Strengthening the Muscular System

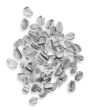

ABOVE *For energy, athletes should eat complex carbohydrates such as nuts.*

FOR THE MUSCLES *to work efficiently we need many of the nervous system nutrients, such as calcium, magnesium, potassium, and sodium – in the correct proportions – for swift passage of messages along the nerves and strong muscle contraction. Additionally, the muscles need a good source of fuel, together with a superb oxygen supply to allow maximum combustion and release of energy. The main foods of the muscles are glycogen and fatty acids, while a good supply of high-quality carbohydrates insures a high level of energy release.*

Exceptional muscular activity also requires a good supply of antioxidant nutrients (to counteract effects of free radicals), iron and zinc (lost in excess sweat), vitamins B6 and C (for adequate repair and maintenance of protein in muscles and collagen), and extra vitamin E, magnesium, and calcium to prevent muscle damage and cramp.

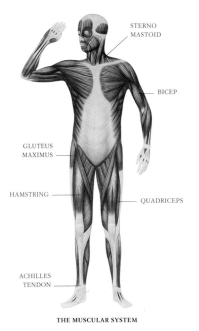

STERNO MASTOID

BICEP

GLUTEUS MAXIMUS

HAMSTRING

QUADRICEPS

ACHILLES TENDON

THE MUSCULAR SYSTEM

IMPROVING ATHLETIC PERFORMANCE

Nutritional considerations
✤ antioxidants (greater rates of oxidation within the body)
✤ calcium and magnesium (for proper muscle function)
✤ potassium together with sodium (needed for proper nerve function)
✤ zinc, iron, and other minerals (to replace those lost in sweat)
✤ vitamin C (for collagen and connective tissue maintenance)
✤ vitamin E (to relieve common muscle cramps)
✤ B vitamins and chromium (to release energy from carbohydrate)
✤ vitamin B6 (for mobilization of protein in muscle growth and repair)
✤ carnitine (needed for fat burning in the muscles)

Maximize
✤ Carbohydrate intake insuring a wide range of complex types including at least half in the form of vegetable carbohydrate, e.g. peas, seed vegetables, pulses (legumes). Also insure you eat plent of ground mixed seeds, especially pumpkin, and antioxidant vegetables and fruit.
Eat
✤ The full quota of fruit for sugar content, a wide range of animal and plant proteins, vegetables and fruit high in potassium (e.g. potatoes, bananas), wheatgerm, molasses, polyunsaturated oils, and olive oil daily.
Avoid
✤ Refined carbohydrate, and minimize intake of dairy food (imbalanced calcium/magnesium), but eat live yogurt daily.

SUGGESTED SUPPLEMENTS

High-potency antioxidant with good levels of betacarotene, vitamins C and E, and selenium; high-potency vitamin B-complex; good-quality multimineral complex containing calcium, magnesium, potassium, zinc, iron, copper, and chromium; essential fatty acids (fish oils, evening primrose oil); L-carnitine; glutamine (to increase lean muscle); Ginseng herb. Take magnesium and potassium after an intensive workout to prevent muscle cramps. Take vitamins B6 and E, calcium, magnesium, potassium, and Aloe vera, to help when muscle cramp occurs.

Disorders of the Endocrine System

ABOVE *Incorporate fruit – such as apricots – into your diet if you are under stress.*

THE ENDOCRINE SYSTEM *relays information around the body by using chemical messengers called hormones. These are produced by glands and are released directly into the bloodstream. The master gland – the pituitary – produces hormones to control the secretions of other endocrine glands, such as the thyroid (which produces thyroxine to regulate the metabolism), and the pancreas (which produces insulin and glucagon to regulate blood-sugar levels).*

Like all body systems, the endocrine system can only work as efficiently as the programing in the genes will allow. Nevertheless, smooth working also depends on receiving the raw materials for its maintenance and from which to synthesize its products. Any suboptimum diet will eventually have an effect on the endocrine system.

By returning to an essentially wholefood diet containing a good supply of essential fatty acids for prostaglandin synthesis, the body starts to receive the basic nutrients it requires to stimulate normal activity of the endocrine glands.

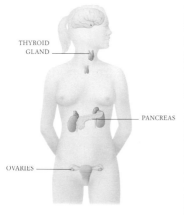

THYROID GLAND

PANCREAS

OVARIES

THE ENDOCRINE SYSTEM

BLOOD-SUGAR PROBLEMS

Nutritional considerations
+ excess refined carbohydrates and sugar
+ excess saturated fat
+ vitamin and mineral deficiencies, or poor absorption
+ excess coffee and alcohol
+ obesity
+ toxicity
+ food intolerance/allergy

Maximize
+ Intake of vegetables and include watercress, Jerusalem artichokes, Brussels sprouts, cucumbers, garlic, and avocado.

Eat
+ Five or six small meals a day, and eat complex carbohydrates regularly (oatmeal, brown rice, etc.).

Avoid
+ All refined and high G.I. foods, additives, sugar, alcohol, caffeine.

SUPPLEMENTS

Multivitamin/multimineral with vitamins A, B-complex, C plus bioflavonoids, and E, magnesium, chromium, zinc, copper, manganese, and potassium; evening primrose oil; lecithin, Aloe vera; lipoic acid.

THYROID IMBALANCE

Nutritional considerations
+ iodine deficiency
+ zinc deficiency
+ selenium deficiency
+ vitamin A deficiency
+ vitamin B6 deficiency
+ vitamin E deficiency
+ excess alcohol
+ fluoride and chlorine contained in tap water
+ overweight/obesity

Maximize
+ Intake of vegetables (especially watercress, radishes, garlic, and seaweed), fruit, mixed seeds (especially linseeds and pumpkin).

Eat
+ Vegetable protein, sprouted seeds, extra wheatgerm or oatgerm. Have one or two Brazil nuts daily.

Avoid
+ Meat, full-fat dairy foods, soy milk, all refined foods, additives, sugar, fatty meats, and alcohol.

SUPPLEMENTS

Multivitamin/multimineral with vitamins A plus betacarotene, B-complex, C, E, zinc, copper, iodine, iron, and selenium; octacosanol (wheatgerm oil); tyrosine (helps nourish thyroid gland).

Disorders of the Digestive System

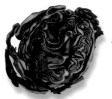

ABOVE *Cabbage and cabbage juice with water are recommended for ulcer sufferers.*

ONE ASPECT OF *nutrition involves understanding how the raw materials from the diet end up as components of the human body. This process starts with the ingestion of food, continues with digestion, and ends with the expulsion of waste material. A wide range of plant and animal materials are broken down into the 50 or so nutrients that our body requires. The choice of foods we eat has an immediate effect on the digestive system – the list of disorders relating to the chewing, digesting, and assimilating of food is endless.*

There are three major areas of digestive problems: poor digestion (low stomach acid and poor digestive enzyme production), food intolerances (undigested food gaining entry to the blood through a "leaky" gut), and poor absorption (accumulated waste material in the large bowel, and the tissues). Therefore, healing the digestive system encompasses not only the introduction of good-quality food but also insures that this good food is going to be digested and absorbed correctly. It is essential to take time to detoxify the system, improve the production of stomach acid and digestive enzymes, and heal the gut lining.

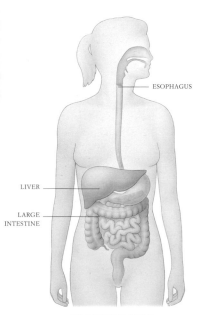

ESOPHAGUS

LIVER

LARGE INTESTINE

THE DIGESTIVE SYSTEM

POOR DIGESTION

Nutritional considerations
✛ food allergy/intolerance
✛ insufficient stomach acid and/or digestive enzymes
✛ poor blood-sugar control
✛ incorrectly combined foods
✛ poor gut flora/presence of gut parasites/overuse of antibiotics
✛ toxic system
✛ low fiber
✛ excess sugars
✛ use of sugar substitute, e.g. aspartame (headaches and migraine)
✛ excess alcohol
✛ excess tea and coffee

Maximize
✛ Intake of antioxidant foods, and fibrous vegetables, pulses (legumes), and rice and barley bran.
Eat
✛ A small pot of live yogurt daily. Add Jerusalem artichokes to your vegetables. Sip a little cider vinegar with meals.
Avoid
✛ All allergenic foods, "rich" foods, and high glycemic index foods. Avoid refined foods, sugar, alcohol, and caffeine. Do not mix concentrated starches and proteins at the same meal.

SUGGESTED SUPPLEMENTS

High-quality multivitamin/multimineral complex containing good levels of vitamins A, B3, B5, B6, B12, folic acid, C and E, calcium, magnesium, selenium, zinc, and potassium; peppermint oil; digestive enzymes (lipase, protease, amylase); betaine hydrochloride; bromelain and papain; Lactobacillus acidophilus; fructo-oligosaccharides; L-glutamine and glucosamine; linseed (flax seed) oil or fish oils.

GALLSTONES

Nutritional considerations
✛ excess cholesterol
✛ excess calcium
✛ excess saturated fat
✛ excess refined food and sugar
✛ low fiber
✛ food allergy/intolerance – may need a hypoallergenic diet
✛ low stomach acid – may need a food combining diet
✛ excess weight

Maximize
✛ Intake of vegetables, seeds, nuts, and pectin-containing foods.

Eat
✛ Foods containing a range of vegetable fiber (cellulose) and minimize cereal fiber. Eat more vegetable protein, such as soy, seed vegetables, pulses (legumes). Sip freshly squeezed lemon juice or cider vinegar with one meal a day. Use olive oil or seed oils daily.

Avoid
✛ Saturated fat, refined foods, common food allergens, dairy foods, sugar, eggs, and pork.

SUPPLEMENTS

Phosphatidyl choline (lecithin); vitamin C taken at maximum level; vitamin E; psyllium seeds or whole linseeds; taurine; ginger.

BELOW *A supplement of whole linseeds can help to treat gallstones.*

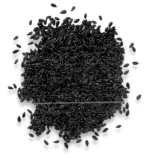

BOWEL DISEASES

Nutritional considerations
✛ many deficiencies (poor absorption)/enzyme insufficiency – may need food combining diet
✛ food allergy/intolerance – may need a hypoallergenic diet
✛ red meat and eggs
✛ refined carbohydrates (e.g. white wheat flour), wheat bran, and sugar
✛ low intake of soluble fiber
✛ fried foods, coffee, spices, salt, and other irritants
✛ aluminum cookware
✛ intestinal parasites/poor gut flora

Maximize
✛ Intake of antioxidant vegetables and fruit, and intake of water and other fluids in between meals. Maximize intake of cellulose fiber and pectins.

Eat
✛ Oily fish and a little chicken, and plant proteins (e.g. tofu).

Avoid
✛ Wheat fiber, all refined food, sugar, coffee, spices, salt, fried red meat, common allergenic foods, additives and aluminum cookware.

SUGGESTED SUPPLEMENTS

Supplements with high levels of vitamins A, B-complex, C, and E, calcium, magnesium, zinc, iron, potassium, and selenium; high-potency garlic; Lactobacillus acidophilus; fructo-oligosaccharides; glucosamine; fish oils and/or linseed (flax seed) oil.

HEARTBURN AND ESOPHAGITIS

Nutritional considerations
✛ excess coffee, alcohol, tea, milk
✛ refined carbohydrates and sugar
✛ saturated and hydrogenated fats, and chocolate
✛ acidic beverages, e.g. orange juice
✛ spicy foods, salt, and additives
✛ drinking liquid with meals (dilutes gastric juices)
✛ excessively hot or cold foods
✛ food allergy/intolerance
✛ eating too quickly or late at night
✛ eating incorrectly combined meals
✛ high or low stomach acid

Eat
✛ Some raw vegetables and sprouted seeds and drink plenty of bottled or filtered tap water in between meals. Have a little Manuka honey. Try and eat five or six small meals a day.

Avoid
✛ Stimulants and acidic foods, and try not to eat hurriedly or late at night. Avoid concentrated carboydrates and proteins at the same meal, saturated and hydrogenated fats, spicy food, spirits, milk, refined carbohydrates, sugar, food additives, food allergens.

SUGGESTED SUPPLEMENTS

High-potency antioxidants; vitamin B-complex, especially B12; vitamin C (as sodium ascorbate if overacid, and ascorbic acid if underacid); bromelain and digestive enzyme complex; glucosamine; silica; Aloe vera; camomile tea; ginger; golden seal; peppermint; slippery elm; cabbage water.

ULCERS (PEPTIC, STOMACH, DUODENAL), HIATUS HERNIA

Nutritional considerations
✤ food intolerance
✤ aspirin
✤ low fiber
✤ wheat fiber
✤ refined carbohydrates and sugar
✤ stimulants (tea, coffee, alcohol, colas, chocolate)
✤ strong spices
✤ excess saturated fat
✤ stomach acid imbalance
Maximize
✤ Intake of cellulose and pectin fiber (omit wheat bran), and all vegetables, fruit, and mixed seeds.
Eat
✤ Manuka honey. Drink cabbage water or juice each day. Take Rooibosh tea.
Avoid
✤ Wheat, wheat bran, alcohol and other stimulants, common allergenic foods, aspirin, saturated fats. Avoid mixing concentrated carbohydrates and proteins at the same meal.

SUPPLEMENTS

Multivitamin/multimineral containing good levels of vitamins A, C, and E, and calcium, magnesium, and zinc; digestive enzymes; deglycyrrhinized licorice; S-methylmethionine; cabbage extract.

LEFT *Increased intake of fresh fruits, such as papaw (papaya), can help with many digestive disorders, such as ulcers and diverticulitis.*

HEPATITIS

Nutritional considerations
✤ alcohol and animal protein
✤ saturated, fried, and hydrogenated oils and fats
✤ refined, low fiber foods
Maximize
✤ Intake of cellulose- and pectin-containing vegetables and fruit and antioxidant vegetables.
Eat
✤ Vegetable protein and fish.
Avoid
✤ Fried and refined food, dairy foods/eggs, sugar, alcohol.

SUPPLEMENTS

Lecithin; psyllium; high-potency antioxidants; Silymarin (Milk thistle); Aloe vera

DIVERTICULITIS

Nutritional considerations
✤ low fiber intake
✤ excess refined carbohydrates
✤ poor bowel flora
Fast
✤ Have a three-day cleanse of steamed vegetables, diluted vegetable juice and/or grape or apple juice, slippery elm tea.
Maximize
✤ Intake of fresh fruit and vegetables. Eat a mixture of vegetable carbohydrates, nuts, pulses, and mixed seeds.

SUPPLEMENTS

Lactobacillus acidophilus; fructo-oligosaccharides; psyllium; vitamins A and C; zinc; ginger; cinnamon; N-acetyl-glucosamine; Aloe vera.

CELIAC DISEASE

Nutritional considerations
✤ gluten intolerance and food allergy/intolerance
✤ vitamin B6 deficiency
✤ digestive enzyme deficiency
Maximize
✤ Freshly ground mixed seeds and nuts.
Eat
✤ A range of vegetable protein, with a little fish and lean meats.
Avoid
✤ All gluten-containing grains (wheats, oats, rye, barley), alcohol.

SUPPLEMENTS

A hypoallergenic multivitamin/multimineral with vitamins A, B-complex, C, D, and E, calcium, magnesium, zinc, and selenium.

ALCOHOLISM

See your physician before embarking on a program
Maximize
✤ Intake of antioxidant vegetables, fruit, and freshly ground mixed seeds.
Eat
✤ Oily fish, live soy yogurt, pulses (legumes), and balanced fiber (cellulose, pectin).
Avoid
✤ Saturated and hydrogenated fat, refined food, sugar, alcohol.

SUPPLEMENTS

A multi-complex containing vitamin B-complex; vitamin E, zinc, selenium, calcium, magnesium; extra vitamin C; L-glutamine.

Disorders of the Excretory System

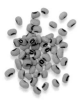

ABOVE *Kidney stone sufferers should eat plenty of pulses such as black-eyed peas.*

THE EXCRETIONS *of waste materials arising from cell metabolism is carried out by the lungs, skin, and the kidneys (which remove nitrogenous waste, used hormones, and so on). A diet that is high in animal protein, animal fat, and refined foods will put an enormous strain on the kidneys, as will a diet with mineral imbalances and an excessive intake of salt. The way to alleviate this stress is to aim for a diet with a good alkali-forming to acid-forming ratio (80 percent alkaline/20 percent acid).*

Using the New Pyramid diet, with gradual change from meat and dairy products to vegetables, pulses (legumes), some wholegrain cereals, and a little fish, will do much to improve the health of this system, increasing the elimination of wastes and reducing the frequency of urinary infections.

KIDNEY STONES

Nutritional considerations
+ excess animal protein and fat
+ excess salt and calcium
+ limited vegetables and fruit
Eat
+ Citrus fruits and alkali-forming vegetables for uric acid stones. Eat more lentils, seed vegetables, and soy. Drink plenty of bottled water in between meals.
Avoid
+ Salt, refined carbohydrates, sugar, coffee, alcohol, red meat, dairy foods.

SUPPLEMENTS

Magnesium citrate/potassium citrate complex; vitamin B6 as pyridoxal-5-phosphate; selenium; cranberry juice/extract.

URINARY TRACT INFECTION

Nutritional considerations
+ low acidity of urine (mineral imbalance)
+ excess sugar
+ low levels of vegetables and fruit
Maximize
+ Antioxidant fruit and vegetables.
Eat
+ Mainly plant protein, with a little oily fish, poultry, and lean meat. Increase fluid intake to around 8 cups (2 liters) a day between meals. Drink cranberry juice between meals.
Avoid
+ Refined foods, especially sugar and alcohol, and minimize intake of dairy foods, especially milk.

SUPPLEMENTS

Concentrated cranberry extract; vitamin C; selenium, fructo-oligosaccharides; Echinacea herb; high-potency garlic; celery seed extract.

NEPHRITIS

Nutritional considerations
+ excess free radicals
+ cow's milk
+ excess animal protein
Maximize
+ Intake of antioxidant fruit and vegetables.
Eat
+ Varied plant protein. Take Manuka honey and goat's milk daily. Drink cranberry juice.
Avoid
+ Cow's milk and other common allergens, red meat, animal protein.

SUPPLEMENTS

High-potency antioxidants, with selenium; vitamin B-complex; vitamin C plus bioflavonoids; magnesium; celery seed extract.

BELOW *Try to replace animal protein with pulses (legumes).*

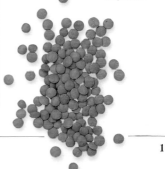

Disorders of the Male Reproductive System

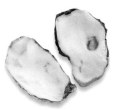

SINCE THIS IS *a book on nutritional healing, it is concerned primarily with correct functioning for cell generation (sperm production) and delivery. Any nutritional help for these areas will also allow nourishment of the brain and the endocrine system, which in turn will improve libido, lift emotions, and remove stress. Again, a basic wholefood diet such as the New Pyramid diet is the place to start. Many of the current problems associated with poor sexual function and infertility are based in poor intake of essential nutrients, but also involve the increasing number of pollutants and estrogens in the environment.*

ABOVE *Oysters may not be aphrodisiacs, but they are good for the prostate and testes.*

Male reproduction problems are mostly focused around the ability to initiate and maintain an erection. Most erectile dysfunction stems from stress and overwork, but where it originates in poor circulation, hormonal imbalance, or overuse of alcohol, nutritional therapy has much to offer.

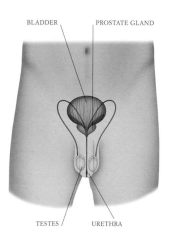

BLADDER

PROSTATE GLAND

TESTES

URETHRA

MALE REPRODUCTIVE ORGANS

PROSTATE ENLARGEMENT

Nutritional considerations
+ alcohol
+ caffeine from tea and coffee
+ low intake of foods containing zinc
+ low intake of antioxidant nutrients
+ excess saturated and hydrogenated fat
+ excess refined foods and sugar
+ low fiber
+ cadmium toxicity – may need a detoxification diet

Maximize
+ Intake of antioxidant fruit and vegetables, especially tomatoes, watermelon, and guava. Insure that you eat plenty of cellulose and pectin fiber along with some cereal fiber.
Eat
+ Oily fish and shellfish (especially oysters), ground mixed seeds (especially pumpkin), and nuts.
Avoid
+ Red meat, full-fat dairy foods, refined carbohydrates, sugar, saturated and hydrogenated fats.
+ Minimize intake of alcohol and caffeine.

SUGGESTED SUPPLEMENTS

Zinc; evening primrose oil; fish oils; amino acids complex – glycine, alanine, and glutamic acid (to help improve urine flow); Saw palmetto; Pygeum africanum.

IMPOTENCE

Nutritional considerations
✢ excess alcohol
✢ excess saturated and hydrogenated fat
✢ excess calcium
✢ excess dairy food
✢ excess refined carbohydrates and sugar
✢ low intake of zinc-rich foods
✢ generalized poor intake of nutrients
✢ excess weight

Maximize
✢ Intake of antioxidant vegetables and fruit, and eat a variety of fibers (cereal, cellulose, pectins). Eat plenty of ground mixed seeds, especially pumpkin seeds.

Eat
✢ Oily fish, shellfish, occasional eggs, soy, pulses (legumes), and seed vegetables as main proteins.

Avoid
✢ Sugar and refined carbohydrates, and minimize intake of animal fats, dairy food, and alcohol.

SUGGESTED SUPPLEMENTS

High-potency vitamin B-complex, with good levels of B3 and B6; zinc; fish oils or linseed (flax seed) oil; Ginkgo biloba; *high-potency garlic.*

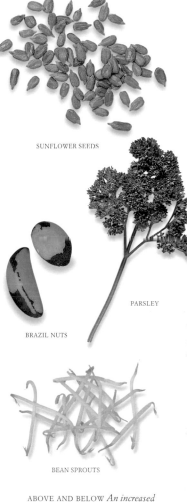

SUNFLOWER SEEDS

PARSLEY

BRAZIL NUTS

MALE INFERTILITY

Nutritional considerations
✢ generalized low intake of essential nutrients
✢ toxicity – may need a detoxification diet
✢ excess refined carbohydrates
✢ excess food additives
✢ excess alcohol

Maximize
✢ Intake of a wide range of vegetables and fruit, eating at least some of them raw, and eat plenty of ground mixed nuts and seeds.

Eat
✢ Sprouted seeds, such as sprouted alfalfa, daily. Minimize animal protein, except for poultry and fish, and eat more soy, beans, and seed vegetables.

Avoid
✢ Refined carbohydrates, artificial additives, alcohol, coffee, tea, fatty meat, non-organic food, and hydrogenated oils.
Wherever possible reduce the levels of environmental toxins, e.g. drink filtered water, do not use plastic containers.

SUGGESTED SUPPLEMENTS

A broad-spectrum multivitamin/multimineral complex, containing good levels of vitamin B-complex, especially B6, B12, and folic acid, vitamin E, iodine, and selenium; vitamin C; zinc; amino acids – especially L-arginine and L-carnitine.

BEAN SPROUTS

ABOVE AND BELOW *An increased intake of raw fruit and vegetables, mixed nuts and seeds, and sprouted seeds may help to counteract male infertility.*

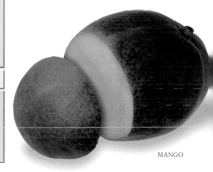

MANGO

Disorders of the Sensory System

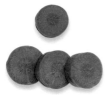

ABOVE *Carotene-rich foods can help with eye problems, such as cataracts.*

WE LIVE IN *a constantly changing environment. Our sense organs allow us to detect these changes, program their usefulness, and then take appropriate action. With our eyes we obtain stereoscopic, wide-angle technicolor vision; with our ears we have stereophonic sound; with our olfactory organs we can detect the faintest odors and with our taste buds tiny differences between sour, sweet, salt, and bitter; with touch we can sense pressure, pain, and pleasure. All these exceptional organs are kept healthy and maintained by vital nutrients.*

A good-quality wholefood diet is essential to supply the necessary raw materials for these activities. In some cases there are special nutrients that are vital to function, such as vitamin A (retinol) for production of "visual purple", the pigment in the retina. More generally, the sensory system is very sensitive to poor peripheral blood flow and the presence of free radicals, so that a diet containing foods that strengthen the fine capillaries and minimize oxidation reactions is essential.

Many infections of the sensory organs, such as conjunctivitis, mouth ulcers, and ear infections, can be prevented by good nutrition that boosts the immune system. Nourishing one part of the body with a good wholefood diet, and nutritional supplements where appropriate, has tremendous effects on all other parts.

CATARACTS

Nutritional considerations
+ excess free radicals
+ low intake of antioxidant nutrients, especially betacarotene, C, and E
+ high intake of saturated fats
+ excess weight
+ milk and other dairy food (lactose)

Maximize
+ Intake of antioxidant vegetables and fruits, especially those rich in carotene, such as carrots and broccoli.
+ Eat plenty of vegetables and fruit rich in vitamin C and freshly ground mixed seeds; and foods high in zinc, e.g. shellfish and pumpkin seeds.

Eat
+ Organic foods where possible. Use a cold-pressed extra virgin olive oil, daily, for vitamin E content.
+ Increase levels of blue/purple fruits and berries.

Avoid
+ Fried, barbecued, and refined foods, saturated and hydrogenated fats, dairy foods, and fatty meats.

SUGGESTED SUPPLEMENTS

Anthocyanidins (grape seed, bilberry, pine bark extract); natural betacarotene; vitamin B2; vitamin C and bioflavonoids; vitamin E; selenium; zinc; Ginkgo biloba; lipoic acid (an antioxidant found in yeast and liver).

RIGHT *A diet high in vital nutrients will keep our hearing, vision, sense of smell, and tastebuds in top condition.*

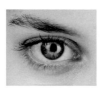

EYES

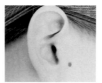

EARS

MOUTH

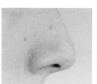

NOSE

NIGHT BLINDNESS

Nutritional considerations
✛ low intake of vitamin A
✛ low levels of antioxidants
✛ excess fat
✛ excess alcohol
Maximize
✛ Intake of antioxidant vegetables
and fruit, especially those
containing betacarotene (carrots,
broccoli, apricots) and
anthocyanidins such as bilberries,
and blueberries.
Eat
✛ Liver once or twice a week (not
if pregnant), plus a little fish –
otherwise keep animal protein at a
low level.
Avoid
✛ Alcohol, artificial sweeteners,
fatty meat, saturated and
hydrogenated fats.

SUPPLEMENTS

*High-potency antioxidants; bilberry
extract; vitamin A; vitamin C; zinc;
Ginkgo biloba; lipoic acid.*

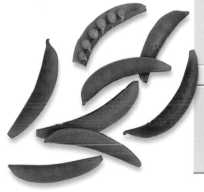

BELOW *A diet high in
antioxidant vegetables, such as
peas, will help with symptoms
of many sight problems.*

CONJUNCTIVITIS

Nutritional considerations
✛ poor nutritional intake
✛ low intake of vitamin C
✛ food intolerance
Maximize
✛ Intake of antioxidant fruit
and vegetables.
Eat
✛ Freshly ground mixed seeds.
✛ Blue/purple berries and fruits.
Avoid
✛ Wheat and dairy products.

SUPPLEMENTS

*Maximum vitamin C, plus
bioflavonoids; zinc; Echinacea herb;
bilberry extract.*

GLAUCOMA

Nutritional considerations
✛ excess meat and dairy products
✛ vitamin and magnesium
deficiency
✛ food intolerance
Maximize
✛ Intake of fresh vegetables and
fruit, and ground mixed seeds.
Avoid
✛ Refined foods, caffeine, sugar,
common allergenic foods, and
alcohol. Minimize intake of meat
and dairy foods.

SUPPLEMENTS

*Anthocyanidins (grape seed,
bilberry); vitamin B-complex, C,
and E; bioflavonoids; natural betacarotene; magnesium; rutin; lipoic
acid, Ginkgo biloba, Aloe vera.*

CORNEAL ULCERS AND RED EYELIDS

Nutritional considerations
✛ low intake of antioxidants
✛ low intake of B vitamins
Maximize
✛ Intake of antioxidant vegetables
and anthocyanidin-containing
berries. Take blackstrap molasses
and oatgerm daily.
Eat
✛ Eat several portions of whole
grains, such as oats, rice, and
millet, each week. Add extra
wheatgerm to cereals, salads, and
soups (unless intolerant to wheat).

SUPPLEMENTS

*High-potency vitamin B-complex,
containing B_3, B_6 and B_5;
vitamin C.*

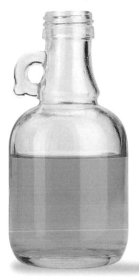

BELOW *Daily use of cold-pressed olive
oil, rich in vitamin E, is recommended
for cataract sufferers.*

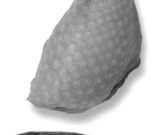

RIGHT *A diet of fruit and vegetables, with a little poutry, is recommended for halitosis sufferers.*

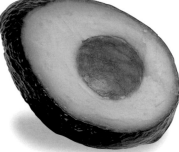

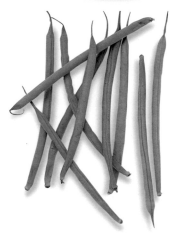

ABOVE *Antioxidant vegetables, such as green beans, can help with tinnitus.*

TINNITUS

Nutritional considerations
✛ food allergy/intolerance
✛ low levels of antioxidants
✛ alcohol
✛ poor calcium/magnesium balance
Maximize
✛ Intake of antioxidant vegetables and fruit.
✛ Drink plenty of filtered or mineral water between meals.
Avoid
✛ Alcohol and common food allergens.

SUPPLEMENTS

High-potency antioxidants; Ginkgo biloba; *zinc; vitamin C.*

INNER EAR DYSFUNCTION

Nutritional considerations
✛ hydrogenated/saturated fats
✛ excess cholesterol and dairy
✛ refined carbohydrates/sugars
Maximize
✛ Antioxidant vegetables, fruit and ground mixed seeds.
Eat
✛ Fibrous and pectin-containing vegetables and oats.
Avoid
✛ Fried foods, sugar, alcohol, coffee.

SUPPLEMENTS

Vitamins A, B-complex, D, C, and E; iron; zinc; ginger; Ginkgo biloba; *Aloe vera.*

HALITOSIS

Nutritional considerations
✛ digestive enzyme deficiency
✛ hydrochloric acid deficiency
✛ food intolerance – may need a hypoallergenic diet
✛ overeating
✛ low fiber
✛ excess animal protein
✛ excess refined carbohydrates
✛ excess dairy foods
✛ toxicity – may need a detoxification diet
✛ candidiasis of the digestive tract

Maximize
✛ Intake of a variety of wholegrains and fiber-rich vegetables and fruit.
Eat
✛ Mainly plant protein (e.g. soy, tofu), with a little fish, poultry, and live yogurt. Eat some raw salad vegetables and sprouted seeds daily. Eat five or six small meals a day and drink at least 8 cups (2 liters) of water. Sip squeezed lemon juice or diluted vinegar with at least two meals daily.
Avoid
✛ Refined carbohydrates, sugar, meat, dairy foods, caffeine, alcohol.

SUGGESTED SUPPLEMENTS

Vitamin A; high-potency vitamin B-complex; vitamin B6 (as pyridoxal-5-phosphate); zinc; digestive enzymes; Lactobacillus acidophilus; *fructo-oligosaccharides; caprilic acid and psyllium (if constipated). Chew any of the following: anise, cardamom, caraway and fennel seeds, parsley, whole cloves, peppermint.*

SISNUSITIS, CATARRH, LOSS OF SMELL

Nutritional considerations
✛ excess dairy foods, starch and sugar
✛ high acid-forming diet
✛ low intake of dark green vegetables
✛ milk allergy
✛ food intolerance – may need a hypoallergenic diet
✛ toxicity (toxemia)
✛ liver congestion – may need a detoxification diet
✛ alcohol
✛ low intake of zinc-rich foods

Maximize
✛ Intake of vegetables (some raw), dark green vegetables, fruit, and ground mixed seeds (pumpkin).
Eat
✛ High-zinc food (fish, shellfish, seaweed) three times a week and increase intake of onions and garlic. Drink fresh vegetable juice daily. Use pulses (legumes) and seed vegetables.
Avoid
✛ Dairy produce, strong spices, common allergens, pork, eggs, alcohol, refined carbohydrates, sugar, and bananas.

SUGGESTED SUPPLEMENTS

Vitamin A; high-potency vitamin B-complex; vitamin C (maximum); high-potency garlic; dandelion herb; Echinacea herb; zinc.

PERIODONTAL DISEASE, MOUTH ULCERS

Nutritional considerations
✛ excess animal protein
✛ saturated and hydrogenated fats
✛ excess gluten, especially wheat
✛ refined carbohydrates and sugar
✛ nutrient deficiencies, especially B vitamins
✛ alcohol
✛ low vegetable fiber and antioxidants
✛ low stomach acid
✛ metal toxicity (amalgam fillings) – may need a detoxification diet
✛ food allergy/intolerance – may need a hypoallergenic diet

Maximize
✛ Intake of antioxidant vegetables and fruit, freshly ground mixed seeds (pumpkin and sesame).
Eat
✛ Oatgerm and/or blackstrap molasses regularly. Increase amount of cellulose and pectin fiber. Eat pulses (legumes), soy, tofu, and seed vegetables. Sip lemon juice or cider vinegar with at least one meal a day.
Avoid
✛ Refined carbohydrates, saturated and hydrogenated fat, sugar, alcohol, additives, red meat, wheat.

SUGGESTED SUPPLEMENTS

High-potency vitamin B-complex, folic acid, vitamin C and bioflavonoids (for wound healing and collagen synthesis); calcium; zinc, coenzyme Q10; Sanguinaria (bloodroot); Aloe vera; Echinacea.

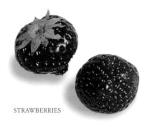
STRAWBERRIES

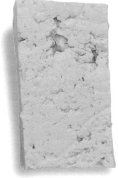
TOFU

ABOVE *Those suffering from periodontal disease and mouth ulcers are advised to eat vegetable protein, such as tofu, and fruit.*

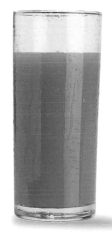

ABOVE *Drink freshly pressed vegetable juice, such as carrot juice, daily to help sinusitis.*

Disorders of the Respiratory System

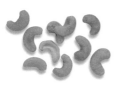

ABOVE *A diet rich in mixed seeds and nuts, such as cashews, can help with hay fever.*

YOU CAN LIVE *weeks without food and four to five days without water, but you can only survive a few minutes without air. The function of the respiratory organs – the lungs, respiratory muscles, and diaphragm – is to provide us with a set of "bellows" to bring oxygen into close contact with the blood supply. This area of close contact has, of necessity, to be moist, delicate, and fragile in order to allow maximum exchange of respiratory gases: oxygen in, and carbon dioxide out. Any disease restricting the intake of air greatly affects general health.*

Serious conditions, such as lung cancer and emphysema, are common, and are usually found in people exposed to air pollution and/or cigarette smoke. Fortunately, in addition to a good basic diet, there are several special nutrients that can help to protect delicate lung membranes from environmental pollutants. Many of these nutrients are antioxidants, which neutralize any free radicals. In addition, the antioxidant nutrients are often useful in boosting the immune system to prevent infections in the respiratory tract. Nutritional therapists also believe that there are some foods, such as dairy food and refined carbohydrates with mucus-generating ability, which can impede the flow of air through these passages. Because the airways are also the first point of contact for any airborne allergens, it is possible to find allergic symptoms in these organs. Cutting out common allergenic foods may help reduce symptoms.

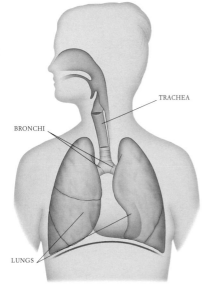

TRACHEA

BRONCHI

LUNGS

THE RESPIRATORY SYSTEM

ASTHMA

Nutritional considerations
✛ excess salt (increases sensitivity to histamine)
✛ food allergy/intolerance – may need a hypoallergenic diet
✛ sulfite sensitivity
✛ dairy foods and wheat
✛ insufficiency of stomach acid – may need a food-combining diet

Maximize
✛ Intake of vegetables and fruit (avoid common allergens, e.g. citrus), and freshly ground mixed seeds, especially pumpkin seeds.

Eat
✛ Mainly vegetable protein such as tofu and beans. Sip diluted cider vinegar with at least one meal a day, and drink plenty of diluted fruit juice or bottled water between meals.

Avoid
✛ Wheat, refined carbohydrates, dairy foods, sugar, salt, sulfured fruits, food additives, and piped water. Keep meat, fish, eggs, coffee, tea, and chocolate to a minimum.

SUGGESTED SUPPLEMENTS

A high-dose multivitamin with B6, and B12; a high-dose multimineral with balanced magnesium and calcium (in 2:1 ratio), and good levels of zinc, molybdenum, and selenium; vitamin C with bioflavonoids; fish oil or linseed (flax seed) oil; Ginkgo biloba extract; anthocyanidins.

BRONCHITIS

Nutritional considerations
✢ excess carbohydrates
✢ acid-forming diet
✢ excess dairy products
✢ vitamin A deficiency
✢ toxic system – may need detoxification diet
✢ food allergy/intolerance – may need a hypoallergenic diet
Maximize
✢ Intake of a good variety of vegetables, fruit, millet, buckwheat, and some pulses (legumes).
Eat
✢ Red-orange vegetables and fruit, such as carrots, bell peppers and apricots, for betacarotene, and eat plenty of ground mixed seeds, especially pumpkin.
Avoid
✢ Refined carbohydrates, sugar, alcohol, dairy produce, common food allergens and "rich" foods. Minimize intake of all grain carbohydrates, animal fat and animal protein.

SUPPLEMENTS

Vitamin A (not if pregnant) and betacarotene; high-potency vitamin B-complex, with B6; vitamin C; high-potency garlic; zinc; Sanguinaria (bloodroot); onion syrup; Aloe vera.

HAY FEVER

Nutritional considerations
✢ food allergy/intolerance – may need hypoallergenic diet
✢ excess carbohydrates, especially refined types
✢ excess sugar
✢ wheat
✢ dairy foods
Maximize
✢ Intake of antioxidant vegetables and fruit, millet, buckwheat, pulses (legumes), and seed vegetables. Eat plenty of ground mixed seeds, especially pumpkin seeds, and nuts.

Avoid
✢ Wheat, refined carbohydrate and sugar, cow's milk, and other common allergenic foods. Minimize intake of grain carbohydrates, animal protein, dairy food, and stimulants (coffee, tea, alcohol, colas).

SUGGESTED SUPPLEMENTS

Vitamin A (as betacarotene if you are pregnant or planning a pregnancy); high-potency B-complex vitamin with B5 and B6; vitamin C plus bioflavonoids; digestive enzymes, containing proteases; zinc; propolis.

BELOW *The respiratory system, from the trachea to the alveoli, is designed to get oxygen to the blood, which then carries it to all the body's cells.*

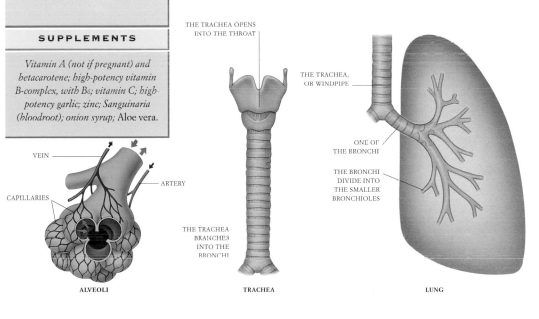

THE TRACHEA OPENS INTO THE THROAT

THE TRACHEA, OR WINDPIPE

ONE OF THE BRONCHI

THE BRONCHI DIVIDE INTO THE SMALLER BRONCHIOLES

VEIN

ARTERY

CAPILLARIES

THE TRACHEA BRANCHES INTO THE BRONCHI

ALVEOLI

TRACHEA

LUNG

Skin, Hair, and Nail Problems

ABOVE *Kiwi fruit, like other fruit high in vitamins, helps alleviate acne.*

THE SKIN IS *the biggest organ we have, and any poor lifestyle or nutritional habits will affect the skin to an enormous extent. A stressful lifestyle, lack of sleep, and a diet low in essential vitamins and minerals will eventually show up in your complexion. Recently, greater emphasis has been placed on treating skin problems from the inside (by nutrition), than by the use of creams and lotions from the outside. A diet of wholefoods and antioxidant-rich vegetables and fruit, will both prevent and heal skin damage.*

The most common agents affecting skin integrity are the free radicals that attack it, both externally from cigarette smoke, pollution, and ultraviolet light, and internally from a diet low in essential nutrients and high in hydrogenated fats, trans-fatty acids, fried food, barbecued food, and highly processed foods. These rogue molecules cause cross-linkage between collagen fibers, and encourage the formation of wrinkles as elasticity decreases. Vitamin C is of particular importance in maintaining a youthful skin since it is an essential nutrient for the formation and maintenance of collagen.

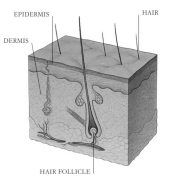

EPIDERMIS

HAIR

DERMIS

HAIR FOLLICLE

THE SKIN

GENERAL SKIN PROBLEMS

Nutritional considerations
✤ stress-generated free radicals requiring treatment with additional nutritional antioxidants
✤ excess refined carbohydrates and sugar
✤ excess saturated and hydrogenated fats
✤ low intake of vegetables and fruit
Maximize
✤ Intake of antioxidant-containing fruit and vegetables, and those containing anthocyanidins, as well as ground mixed seeds.
Eat
✤ A good balanced mixture of wholegrain carbohydrates and vegetable carbohydrates, and insure you have some raw vegetables and sprouted seeds and pulses (legumes) every day.

Avoid
✤ Refined carbohydrates, sugar, saturated and hydrogenated fat, alcohol, food additives, polluted food, unfiltered piped water, and common allergenic foods. Minimize intake of red meat, fatty meat, and dairy products, and consume mainly vegetable protein, such as tofu and pulses (legumes), with a little oily fish, poultry and occasional eggs.

SUGGESTED SUPPLEMENTS

High-potency antioxidant formula; extra vitamins C and E (vitamin E, together with zinc, helps with stretch marks); anthocyanidins (bilberry, etc.); evening primrose oil (for dry skin); high-potency B-complex vitamins (for an oily skin); iron (useful for itchy skin); lysine for cold sores; application of Aloe vera *gel.*

SUNBURN

Follow the New Pyramid diet.

SUPPLEMENTS

Use for two or three weeks before exposure to sun: vitamin E, beta-carotene, vitamin C, selenium. Treat burns with Aloe vera or tea-tree oil.

ACNE

Nutritional considerations
+ poor gut flora (overuse of antibiotics)
+ excess saturated fats and fried foods
+ low fiber
+ excess refined carbohydrates and sugar
+ dairy foods
+ food intolerance, especially to chocolate, some nuts, and cola drinks – may need to follow a hypoallergenic diet
Maximize
+ Intake of antioxidant nutrients, and mixed seeds, especially pumpkin seeds.
Eat
+ Live yogurt daily. Increase intake of soluble fibers (fruit and vegetables).
Avoid
+ Refined carbohydrates, common allergenic foods, dairy (except yogurt), and fried foods. Minimize saturated fat.

SUPPLEMENTS

High-potency multivitamin/multi-mineral containing good levels of vitamins A, B6, C, and E, selenium, zinc, and chromium.

BODY ODOR

Nutritional considerations
+ excess saturated fats and hydrogenated fats
+ meat, dairy, fried foods
+ toxicity
+ low intake of zinc-rich foods. and essential fatty acids
Maximize
+ Intake of ground seeds, especially pumpkin seeds.
Eat
+ Organic produce and shellfish, fish, and nuts several times a week.

SUPPLEMENTS

A colon and liver cleanse complex; magnesium; zinc; fish oils or linseed oil; evening primrose oil; lecithin.

HIVES

Nutritional considerations
+ chlorine in drinking water
+ toxicity – may need to follow a detoxification diet
+ food allergy/intolerance – commonly shellfish, milk, eggs, wheat, pork, onions, some fruit – may need a hypoallergenic diet
+ stomach acid deficiency – may need food-combining diet
+ food additives (color and preservatives)
+ coffee
+ alcohol

Maximize
+ Intake of freshly ground mixed seeds, especially pumpkin seeds.
Eat
+ Oily fish (herring, mackerel, salmon) and vegetable protein (soy) instead of meat, poultry, and dairy proteins. Sip diluted cider vinegar with main meal and drink bottled water between meals.
Avoid
+ Saturated fat, hydrogenated fat, refined foods, food additives, coffee, chlorinated water, all allergens above, and alcohol.

SUGGESTED SUPPLEMENTS

Vitamin A; vitamin B-complex (especially with B6 and B12), vitamin C; calcium.

ECZEMA

Nutritional considerations
+ food allergy/intolerance (cow's milk, eggs, wheat, red meat, sugar, tea, coffee, and alcohol)
+ low stomach acid
Maximize
+ Intake of ground seeds, especially pumpkin.
Eat
+ Tofu and vegetable proteins, and some oily fish. Drink bottled water.
Avoid
+ Saturated/hydrogenated fat, refined food, allergens (see above).

SUPPLEMENTS

Evening primrose oil; fish oil or linseed (flax seed) oil; multiformula with zinc, vitamins A and C.

PSORIASIS

Nutritional considerations
✛ low fiber
✛ excess meat
✛ possible copper-induced deficiency of zinc.
✛ food allergy/intolerance – may need a hypoallergenic diet
✛ poor acid/alkaline balance
✛ low intake of essential fatty acids
✛ suboptimum liver function – may need a detoxification diet
Maximize
✛ Intake of alkali-forming vegetables and fruit, freshly ground mixed seeds, especially pumpkin seeds, and vegetable fiber and pectin (e.g. apples and carrots).
Eat
✛ At least some raw vegetables daily. Concentrate on brown rice, millet, and buckwheat as main cereals. Drink filtered water or bottled mineral water.
Avoid
✛ Citrus fruit, tomatoes, red meat, saturated fats, hydrogenated fats, candy, alcohol, and refined carbohydrates.
✛ Minimize intake of animal protein (except oily fish and shellfish); use soy and pulses (legumes).

SUGGESTED SUPPLEMENTS

A high-potency antioxidant formula including zinc and selenium; Milk thistle herb; magnesium fumarate; B-complex vitamins; linseed (flax seed) oil; fish oils; Aloe vera juice; herbal colon cleanse; lipase.

IMPETIGO

Nutritional considerations
✛ toxicity – may need a detoxification diet
✛ low intake of protein
✛ excess sweet food and fruits
✛ excess acidity
✛ low intake of dark green vegetables.
✛ dairy foods
Maximize
✛ Intake of dark green vegetables and freshly ground mixed seeds, especially pumpkin.
Eat
✛ Mainly plant protein such as soy, pulses (legumes), and seed vegetables, with a little oily fish.
✛ Aim for an 80 percent alkaline to 20 percent acid diet.
Avoid
✛ Alcohol, sugar, refined carbohydrate, saturated and hydrogenated fats, meat, and dairy foods. Minimize intake of sweet fruit and honey.

SUGGESTED SUPPLEMENTS

Vitamins A and C; high-potency garlic; zinc; essential fatty acids (fish oils/ linseed (flax seed) oil, and evening primrose/starflower oil); golden seal herb; tea-tree oil for external application.

ROSACEA (ACNE ROSACEA)

Nutritional considerations
✛ alcohol, coffee, tea, spices
✛ low levels of stomach acid and digestive enzymes
✛ low intake of B vitamins
Maximize
✛ Intake of freshly ground mixed seeds (pumpkin) and antioxidant vegetables and fruit.
Eat
✛ At least some raw vegetables and sprouted seeds daily.

SUPPLEMENTS

Betaine hydrochloride; digestive enzymes; high-potency vitamin B-complex; zinc; fructo-oligosaccharides.

WARTS AND VERRUCAE

Nutritional considerations
✛ low intake of nutrient-dense foods
✛ low intake of vitamin A
Maximize
✛ Intake of antioxidant fruit and vegetables, and sea vegetables, as well as seeds (especially pumpkin).
Eat
✛ Plenty of zinc-containing foods (fish, shellfish, pulses (legumes), raw vegetables, and sprouted seeds.

SUPPLEMENTS

High-potency antioxidant formula containing good levels of vitamins A (as betacarotene if you are pregnant or planning to become pregnant) and C, selenium, and zinc.

DANDRUFF

Nutritional considerations
+ acid diet
+ excess carbohydrates and sugar
+ excess alcohol and salt
+ excess citrus
+ low intake of dark green vegetables
+ excess saturated fats and hydrogenated fats
+ food allergy/intolerance, especially to wheat and dairy foods
+ low intake of essential fatty acids
+ low intake of foods containing vitamins A, B-complex, E, and zinc
+ low activity of digestive enzymes

Maximize
+ Intake of orange and dark green vegetables and antioxidant fruit (except citrus) and vegetables. Eat plenty of ground seeds (especially pumpkin) nuts, oatgerm, and avocado.

Eat
+ Some raw vegetables and sprouted seeds daily. Increase amount of fish, shellfish, and pulses (legumes).

Avoid
+ Refined food, saturated and hydrogenated fats, alcohol, salt, sugar, citrus, wheat, dairy foods, allergens. Minimize grain carbohydrates.

SUGGESTED SUPPLEMENTS

Vitamin A (as betacarotene if pregnant); vitamin B-complex (with B6, B12, and folic acid); evening primrose oil; zinc; digestive enzymes; lecithin.

DULL, DRY, OR LUSTERLESS HAIR

Nutritional considerations
·+ low intake of vitamin A, protein, and essential fatty acids
+ excess refined carbohydrates and saturated fats

Maximize
+ Intake of vitamin A-containing vegetables and fruit (carrots, apricots, mango, broccoli), as well as mixed seeds.

Eat
+ Plenty of fish, soy, pulses (legumes), and lean meat for protein.

Avoid
+ Refined carbohydrates and saturated fats.

SUGGESTED SUPPLEMENTS

Fish oils, linseed (flax seed) oil, and evening primrose oil, or starflower oil; zinc; vitamin B-complex; Aloe vera; Ginkgo biloba.

BALDNESS (ALOPECIA), HAIR LOSS

Nutritional considerations
+ poor nutrition of the glandular system, especially the thyroid, adrenals, and pituitary
+ single or multiple deficiencies of vitamin B complex, especially B6, biotin, folic acid, inositol, and P.A.B.A. (para-aminobenzoic acid)
+ refined food, especially sugar
+ alcohol and nicotine
+ heavy metal poisoning – may need a detoxification diet
+ foods low in antioxidants
+ crash and "yo-yo" dieting

Maximize
+ Intake of antioxidant-containing fruit and vegetables, and ground mixed seeds.

Eat
+ Added wheatgerm on salads and soups, and take blackstrap molasses daily. Eat oily fish and lean meat in balance with soy products and pulses (legumes).

Avoid
+ All refined food, sugar, food additives, polluted food (eat organic), and alcohol.

SUPPLEMENTS

A high-potency multivitamin/multi-mineral containing good levels of vitamins A, C, B (especially B3, B5, B6, B12 and P.A.B.A., biotin, and folic acid) and E, and iron, zinc, and selenium; iodine; lecithin.

ABOVE *A diet rich in pumpkin seeds can help restore luster to dull or dry hair.*

The Female Reproductive System

THERE ARE VARIOUS *ailments that only apply to women. Breast disease, P.M.S., menstrual abnormalities, fibroids, endometriosis, and female infertility are prevalent among women of menstruating age. Postmenopausal women also suffer from a similar number of ailments associated with the winding down of the female reproductive process, but additionally, the effects on health can be more widespread, resulting in conditions such as osteoporosis and circulatory disorders.*

ABOVE *For inflammation of the fallopian tubes eat plenty of seeds and vegetable protein.*

BREAST TISSUE

The mammary or breast tissue is composed of secretory cells and ducts. The ducts of the breast branch through the breast tissue and are connected to glands called the alveoli, which secrete breast milk. A number of hormones stimulate breast development during pregnancy and menstruation. Under the influence of these hormones, the breasts increase in size, and the ductal system and alveolar structures become more complex.

The periodic stimulation of the breasts by menstruation and pregnancy can lead to breast disease. At least 20 percent of premenopausal women have non-cancerous lumpy, tender breasts, often the result of fibrocystic breast disease. The condition may be stable, or may worsen before menstruation. The more fat in the diet, the greater the risk of benign breast disease.

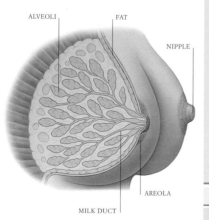

ALVEOLI   FAT

NIPPLE

AREOLA

MILK DUCT

ABOVE *Breast milk is created in the alveoli, and is conducted to the nipple through ducts.*

BREAST CANCER

Nutritional considerations
+ low fiber intake
+ obesity
+ excess saturated and hydrogenated fats and trans-fatty acids
+ excess animal protein/dairy foods
+ excess refined carbohydrates and sugar
+ xeno-estrogens in water and food
+ estrogen dominance (from use of the contraceptive pill and/or hormone replacement therapy)
+ low intake of antioxidants
+ suboptimum liver activity

Maximize
+ Intake of antioxidant fruit and vegetables, and mixed seeds.
Eat
+ Foods containing phytoestrogens (tofu, tempeh, miso, celery, fennel, rhubarb, oats, rye) and anti-cancer nutrients (cabbage, sprouts, cauliflower, broccoli). Eat a pot of live soy yogurt daily and use cold-pressed virgin olive oil daily.
Avoid
+ Saturated and hydrogenated fats, refined carbohydrates, and sugar.

SUGGESTED SUPPLEMENTS

A good-quality multivitamin/multimineral formula; high doses of vitamin C; an antioxidant formula containing good levels of selenium, zinc, and lipoic acid; chromium; Lactobacillus acidophilus; coenzyme Q10; Siberian ginseng; wild yam extract.

BENIGN AND FIBROCYSTIC BREAST DISEASE

Nutritional considerations
✢ processed foods
✢ excess saturated fat
✢ excess dairy foods
✢ excess refined carbohydrates
✢ low intake of vitamins (especially vitamin E) and minerals (selenium and iodine)
✢ presence of methylanthines – caffeine and theobromine – in coffee, chocolate, cola beverages, some teas, and some drugs
✢ food allergy/intolerance
✢ estrogen excess/hormonal imbalance
Maximize
✢ Intake of antioxidant vegetables and fruit, sea vegetables, seeds, and nuts.
Eat
✢ Wheat-or oatgerm on salads and soups, use olive oil along with other seed oils (sesame, sunflower) on salads. Drink bottled/mineral water between meals and eat live yogurt daily.
Avoid
✢ Refined carbohydrates, saturated and hydrogenated fats, trans-fatty acids, methylxanthines, additives, pesticides, and common allergens. Minimize dairy foods and avoid plastic food containers.

SUPPLEMENTS

High-potency multivitamin formula containing vitamins A (as betacarotene if pregnant or planning a pregnancy), B (especially B₁ and B₆), C, and E; balanced calcium/ magnesium formula; selenium; evening primrose oil or starflower (borage) oil; fish oils or linseed (flax seed) oil; kelp, or iodized salt.

THE CERVIX

The cervix, uterus, fallopian tubes, and vagina play a vital part in conception and pregnancy. If nutrition is poor, these organs can become damaged. The ovarian tissue can become fibrous and give rise to cysts or, occasionally, ovarian cancer; and the cervix can become damaged, leading to abnormal cell growth.

The cervix is the lower tip of the uterus that extends into the vagina. Any abnormal cell development (cervical dysplasia) picked up in a routine "smear" test is a cause of concern. Fortunately, effective treatment can prevent the development of cervical cancer, and a wholesome diet and healthy lifestyle will complement any medical treatment.

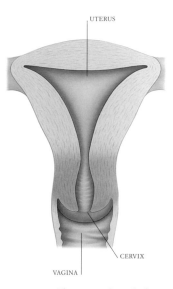

ABOVE *The cervix is the neck of the uterus and protrudes into the upper section of the vagina.*

CERVICAL AND OVARIAN PROBLEMS

Nutritional considerations
✢ excess animal protein
✢ stimulants (tea, coffee, sugar, salt)
✢ excess alcohol
✢ refined and overcooked foods
✢ contraceptive pill (encourages folic acid deficiency)
✢ deficient intake of fresh fruit and vegetables
Maximize
✢ Intake of antioxidant and phytochemical-containing vegetables and fruit.

Eat
✢ A diet that balances animal protein (fish only) with vegetable protein (seeds, nuts, beans, and tofu). Eat at least some vegetables raw, wheatgerm and sprouted seeds daily. Drink fresh carrot, or other vegetable, juice daily.
Avoid
✢ Tea, coffee, alcohol, salt, sugar, refined carbohydrates, saturated and hydrogenated fats and trans-fatty acids, wheat, processsed food, food additives, and common food allergens.

SUGGESTED SUPPLEMENTS

A high-potency antioxidant formula containing good levels of beta-carotene, vitamin C, and selenium; a high-potency vitamin B-complex containing good levels of B₁₂ and folic acid.

THE VAGINA

Many harmless micro-organisms are normally found in the vagina, and they consist of a very large number of yeasts and bacteria. Some of these coexisting organisms are essential to normal vaginal health, such as certain species of *Lactobacillus*. The diversity of vaginal flora is controlled by several factors. The most important of these is the amount of glucose present in vaginal secretions, the acid/alkali balance of the body, and the hormonal state.

Diets high in refined carbohydrates and sugar, especially when hormonal imbalance is present, will tend to allow overgrowths of unfavorable microbes. Antibiotics kill pathogenic bacteria and helpful acid-producing bacteria indiscriminately, preventing natural control of pathogenic bacteria and yeasts.

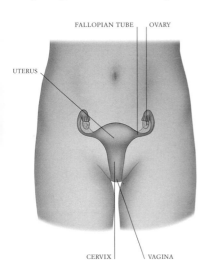

FALLOPIAN TUBE OVARY

UTERUS

CERVIX VAGINA

ABOVE *The female reproductive system is both complex and finely tuned; fortunately, the majority of problems that can occur respond well to treatment with nutrition.*

VAGINITIS

Nutritional considerations
✢ damaged gut ecology (dysbiosis), by antibiotics
✢ contraceptive pill (causing pH changes and possible vitamin B6 deficiency)
✢ blood sugar problems
✢ low intake of vitamin B-complex, especially B6
✢ excess refined carbohydrates and sugar
✢ low intake of antioxidant nutrients (needed for neutralizing stress-induced free radicals)
✢ food allergy/intolerance – may need a hypoallergenic diet
Maximize
✢ Intake of antioxidant-containing vegetables, vegetable protein, seeds, nuts, soy, pulses (legumes), and seed vegetables.
Eat
✢ A high-alkali-forming diet. Take care with excess fruit – avoid sweet and dried fruit. Add wheatgerm or oatgerm to cereals, salads, and soups. Eat five or six small meals a day, each containing a little protein, and eat one small pot of live soy yogurt daily.
Avoid
✢ Refined carbohydrates, sugar, alcohol, yeast-containing foods (e.g. vinegar, wine, pickles, etc.) and common food allergens.

SUPPLEMENTS

A high-quality multivitamin/ multimineral complex, containing good levels of vitamins A (as beta-carotene if pregnant), B-complex (especially B6), C, E, and zinc; high-potency garlic; Lactobacillus acidophilus; grapefruit seed extract; fructo-oligosaccharides. Treat the affected area with plain live yogurt.

THE FALLOPIAN TUBES AND UTERUS

The fallopian tubes (and ovaries) are open to the outside world – with all its foreign infective agents – via the vagina and uterus. However, these delicate inner passageways and glands are protected by in built self-defense mechanisms and barriers. The vagina, being normally acidic, prevents pathogens from flourishing; the thick mucous plug of the cervix acts as a mechanical barrier to any invading bodies; and hairlike cilia in the uterus and fallopian tubes constantly waft any debris or bacteria back down toward the cervix and vagina. However, these protective measures fail during menstruation, when the vagina becomes relatively alkaline and the cervical plug is removed. Fortunately, a healthy menstrual flow will usually prevent infection getting through.

A copper I.U.D. can also be a major cause of problems, due either to infection at the time of insertion or to mechanical irritation and congestion, which creates a more favorable environment for bacterial growth. An I.U.D. may also increase the amount of copper in the body, which can lead to low levels of zinc. Suboptimum nutrition, especially if immune-boosting nutrients are minimal, can allow these conditions to continue. Nutritional therapists think a mucus-forming diet (excess animal products, especially dairy foods, and excess carbohydrate) can thicken the fluids in the fallopian tubes, causing blockages. Making these dietary changes may allow clearing of the blockage and removal of the infectious agents.

ENDOMETRIOSIS

This is a condition in which the womb lining (endometrium) grows in sites outside the uterus (in the ovaries, fallopian tubes, ligaments, bowel, or bladder). This tissue responds to the natural hormone cycle and sheds blood within these body cavities, often causing inflammation, pain, and in extreme cases, infertility. Symptoms include pain on ovulation, pain during or after sexual intercourse, heavy or irregular bleeding, depression, painful bowel and bladder movements, and intestinal upsets. It is important to seek a proper medical diagnosis before embarking on any self-help measures or nutritional programs.

Nutritional considerations
✢ low nutrient intake or poor absorption
✢ excess animal protein/animal fat
✢ gut dysbiosis
✢ food allergy/intolerance

Balance
✢ Animal proteins (fish only) with plant proteins (seeds, nuts, soy, pulses [legumes], and seed vegetables).

Eat
✢ Two helpings of dark green leafy vegetables and a pot of live soy yogurt daily. Sip diluted lemon juice or cider vinegar with the main meal.

Avoid
✢ Animal fats, dairy foods, red meat, refined foods, and common allergens.

SUGGESTED SUPPLEMENTS

A high-potency vitamin/multimineral formula containing good levels of all the major nutrients and especially vitamin B-complex, vitamin C, and the minerals magnesium, zinc, and selenium; an additional magnesium/calcium balanced complex; DL-phenylalanine (as a natural painkiller); probiotics and digestive enzymes; evening primrose and fish oils.

SALPINGITIS AND SALPINGO-OOPHORITIS

Salpingitis (inflammation and congestion of the fallopian tubes) and salpingo-oophoritis (inflammation of the ovaries) are rare conditions.

Nutritional considerations
✢ excess carbohydrates
✢ excess sugar
✢ excess dairy products
✢ low intake of immune-boosting nutrients

Maximize
✢ Intake of antioxidant fruit and vegetables, seeds, and vegetable protein.

Eat
✢ Oily fish twice a week and limit the amount of wholegrain carbohydrates that you consume.

SUPPLEMENTS

A high-potency antioxidant containing good levels of vitamins A (as betacarotene if you could be pregnant), C, E, and selenium and zinc; golden seal (unless pregnant); saw palmetto; wild yam extract.

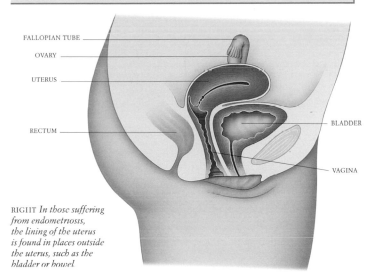

FALLOPIAN TUBE
OVARY
UTERUS
RECTUM
BLADDER
VAGINA

RIGHT *In those suffering from endometriosis, the lining of the uterus is found in places outside the uterus, such as the bladder or bowel.*

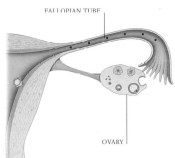

FALLOPIAN TUBE
OVARY

ABOVE *The ovaries produce eggs. After an egg is fertilized in the fallopian tubes it travels to the uterus, where the fetus develops.*

MENSTRUATION

The first consideration in dealing with menstrual disorders is always to look for any disease that may be the cause. Any bleeding between periods should be investigated by your physician for possible cancer, fibroids, or cervical lesions. However, menstrual problems are most likely to be caused by hormonal imbalances, and various tests can be undertaken to assess the levels of F.S.H. and L.H. (pituitary hormones controlling the menstrual cycle). Hormone production and regulation are affected by stress, so any lifestyle problems need to be addressed.

The entire hormonal balance that governs the menstrual cycle can be upset by taking the contraceptive pill, extreme diets, very strict weight-loss regimes, or excessive exercise. Redress the balance through optimum nutrition.

MENSTRUAL DISORDERS

Nutritional considerations
✢ excess refined food
✢ excess intake of stimulants (coffee, tea, colas, salt, sugar)
✢ excess intake of animal protein and animal fat
✢ low intake or poor absorption of calcium and magnesium
✢ generalized nutritional deficiencies
✢ hormonal imbalance (sometimes due to excessive exercise and/or stress)
✢ toxicity – may need a detoxification diet
✢ excess alcohol

Maximize
✢ Intake of a wide range of fruit and vegetables, especially dark green vegetables, and freshly ground mixed seeds, especially sesame and pumpkin.

Eat
✢ Oily fish and lean meat, and balance with vegetable proteins. Have five or six small meals a day, eating a small amount of protein to balance the carbohydrate at each meal.

Avoid
✢ Refined foods, coffee, salt, sugar, and alcohol.

SUGGESTED SUPPLEMENTS

A multivitamin/multimineral formula with good levels of vitamins A (betacarotene if contemplating pregnancy), B-complex (especially B3, and B6), C, D, and E, and calcium, magnesium, iron, and zinc (or take iron as a separate supplement); anthocyanidins (bilberry extract, etc.) – especially for dysmenorrhea and bloating; lecithin; high-potency garlic; kelp; evening primrose oil or starflower oil; fish oils; protein (aminoacid) complex; digestive enzymes; wild yam extracts.

NUTRITIONAL LEVELS AFFECTED BY THE PILL

The contraceptive pill can upset the hormonal balance of the body, and consequently can have a profound effect on the nutrients the body needs and how it treats those that are absorbed.

NUTRIENT	INFLUENCE OF THE PILL	NUTRIENT	INFLUENCE OF THE PILL
Vitamin A	Increases circulating levels of vitamin A, prudent to stop taking the pill at least three months before trying to conceive.		supplementing with folic acid for several months before trying to conceive is important (see page 127).
Vitamin B1	Increases requirements for this vitamin.	**Vitamin C**	Increases requirement for vitamin C, but
Vitamin B2	Increases requirements for this vitamin.		avoid taking more than 1,000mg per day –
Vitamin B6	Alters vitamin B6 status and this may be linked to depression, impaired glucose tolerance, poor digestion, and increased		excess vitamin C may change a low-dose estrogen pill to a high-dose one, and increase the adverse effects of the pill.
	risk of cancer of the urinary tract.	**Copper**	Increases serum copper levels.
Vitamin B12	Adversely influences levels of B12. May be	**Iron**	Lowers serum iron in some women, but in
	related to psychiatric symptoms.		others iron status may increase.
Folic Acid	Possibly interferes with blood cell	**Magnesium**	Possibly lowers levels of magnesium.
	formation. Deficiency is now closely linked	**Zinc**	Lowers plasma zinc – possibly because of
	to neural tube abnormalities in babies, so		high copper levels.

PREMENSTRUAL SYNDROME

P.M.S. is very widespread, affecting one in three menstruating women. It can also be very serious; the hormonal deficiency of progesterone that often accompanies P.M.S. has been shown to increase the risk of breast cancer. The psychological effects may occasionally be extreme enough to make women feel suicidal or violent/aggressive. The symptoms can be many and varied; they include radical mood swings, tender breasts, acne, fluid retention, weight gain, cravings and binge eating, insomnia, crying, dizziness, fainting, headaches, palpitations, confusion, lethargy, abdominal bloating, depression, anxiety, and fatigue.

Although P.M.S. is widespread in the Western world, it is actually quite uncommon in more traditional societies, and this suggests that diet and lifestyle play a large part in the problem. P.M.S. is associated with an increased intake of refined carbohydrates and, specifically, a greatly increased intake of sugar. Since carbohydrates enhance mood by the synthesis of serotonin (a neurotransmitter), women feeling anxious and depressed often increase their intake of these substances. But large amounts of sweet food can cause fluid retention, hypoglycemic symptoms, and loss of magnesium.

RIGHT *Some women experience emotional as well as physical symptoms with P.M.S. Eating green and raw vegetables relieves these symtoms.*

PREMENSTRUAL SYNDROME (P.M.S.)

Nutritional considerations
✛ excess animal fat/dairy products
✛ excess sugar and refined carbohydrates
✛ stimulants (tea, coffee, chocolate, colas, alcohol, salt, caffeine)
✛ generalized low intake (or poor absorption) of nutrients
✛ estrogen dominance/xeno-estrogens
✛ poor levels of digestive enzymes
✛ low intake of foods high in magnesium, e.g. seeds
✛ difficulty metabolizing linoleic acid
✛ essential fatty acid deficiency
✛ lead toxicity

Maximize
✛ Intake of fruit and vegetables, especially dark green vegetables such as cabbage and broccoli, as well as ground seeds (sunflower, sesame, pumpkin, linseed).
Eat
✛ Fish, poultry, pulses (legumes) as your main source of protein. Eat some raw vegetables and sprouted beans daily. Eat five or six small meals a day. Soy yogurt and fruit should satisfy craving for sweet foods.
Avoid
✛ Alcohol, refined carbohydrates, sugar, salt, hydrogenated and saturated fats, trans-fatty acids.

SUGGESTED SUPPLEMENTS

A high-potency multivitamin/multimineral complex containing good levels of vitamin B-complex (especially B3, B6, and biotin), vitamin C, and the minerals and magnesium, calcium, all trace elements (especially zinc and chromium); an additional balanced calcium/magnesium complex may be required; evening primrose oil or starflower (borage) oil; fish oils; vitamin E (especially for breast tenderness); fructo-oligosaccharides; L-methionine; L-tyrosine ; wild yam extract; Dong quai; Milk thistle; Ginkgo biloba; digestive enzymes.

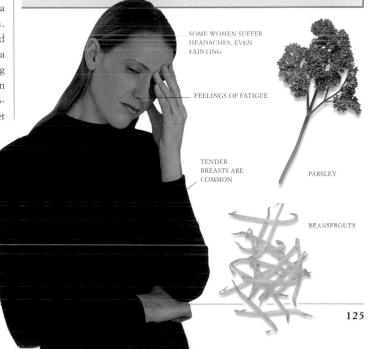

SOME WOMEN SUFFER HEADACHES, EVEN FAINTING

FEELINGS OF FATIGUE

TENDER BREASTS ARE COMMON

PARSLEY

BEANSPROUTS

Fertility

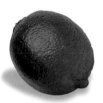

ABOVE *Antioxidant fruit, including limes, boost immunity and increase chances of pregnancy.*

THERE ARE MANY *physical and medical causes of infertility outside the scope of this book. In general, however, women who wish to become pregnant for the first time are more likely to succeed if they regulate their diet so that they are neither excessively underweight nor overweight. Studies show that around 12 percent of women who are infertile for ovulatory reasons are equally divided between being overweight and underweight.*

INFERTILITY AND RECURRENT MISCARRIAGE

Miscarriage can happen to any woman because of a chance event or some ongoing stressful condition, but recurrent miscarriages (three or more) are a different matter. There are many and varied causes and they should be investigated thoroughly by a gynecologist. Miscarriages can be caused by nutritional deficiencies, hormone imbalance, diabetes, thyroid problems, anatomical problems with the womb, fibroids, chromosomal abnormalities, and infections such as chlamydia and herpes. Fertility can be reduced by alcohol and nutrient deficiencies.

BELOW *Antioxidant vegetables, such as celery, can boost your fertility.*

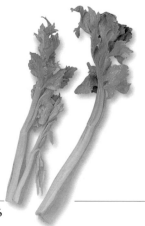

FACTORS AFFECTING FERTILITY

Nutritional considerations
✛ low levels of body fat
✛ excessive slimming and/or excessive exercise
✛ obesity
✛ alcohol and caffeine
✛ imbalance of vitamin A
✛ low intake (or poor absorption) of B vitamins, especially B6
✛ toxicity and acidity
✛ excess animal protein and fat
Maximize
✛ Intake of immune-boosting fruit and vegetables, seeds and nuts.
Eat
✛ Eat mostly vegetable protein with a little fish and lean meat. Add wheatgerm or oatgerm to salads. Increase foods high in betacarotene (carrots, apricots).
Avoid
✛ Red meat, refined foods, alcohol.

SUPPLEMENTS

A good-quality multivitamin/ multimineral complex containing betacarotene, vitamin B-complex (especially B6, B12, and folic acid), and E and zinc; evening primrose or starflower (borage) oil, and fish oils.

DEFICIENCIES LINKED WITH MISCARRIAGE

Nutritional considerations
✛ toxicity
✛ excess refined carbohydrates
✛ artificial additives
✛ alcohol
✛ generalized vitamin and mineral deficiencies
Maximize
✛ Intake of antioxidant fruit and vegetables, and freshly ground mixed seeds (sunflower, pumpkin, sesame, and linseed [flax seed]).
Balance
✛ Animal protein (fish, poultry, and some free-range eggs) with plant proteins. Take fiber in a variety of forms: oats, brown rice, cellulose, pectins.
Avoid
✛ Refined carbohydrates, sugar, additives, alcohol and other stimulants, liver, pesticides in food.

SUPPLEMENTS

A good-quality multivitamin/ multimineral complex with good levels of the B-complex, betacarotene, vitamin E, zinc, selenium, manganese; evening primrose oil or starflower (borage) oil and fish oils.

PRECONCEPTUAL CARE

The nutritional status of the father and mother in the weeks and months before conception can influence the outcome of a pregnancy. Excessive intake of toxic metals (lead, cadmium, and mercury) can affect the quality of the sperm, and smoking and alcohol can increase the number of sperm abnormalities and lower overall sperm count.

Genetic damage can be made worse by nutritional deficiencies of, for example, folic acid, B-vitamin complex, vitamins C, E, and zinc. Excessive amounts of vitamin A, on the other hand, can lead to congenital abnormalities. Neural tube defects (such as spina bifida) have been strongly linked to inadequate levels of folic acid in the mother's diet. It is likely that the lack of other nutrients is also related to this type of birth defect.

If the woman's diet has been poor or at very best suboptimum prior to conception, then there will not be the required levels of nutrients available for the initial development of the fetus, even if the new mother embarks upon a better diet. Any nutrient deficiencies need to be rectified before conception – changes in diet and lifestyle aimed at increasing the likelihood of conception should ideally be made at least three months before the intended time.

Most pregnant women have a normal healthy baby even without a preconceptual program of optimum nutrition and lifestyle changes. The recommendations on this page are for women who are not yet pregnant and who want to maximize their level of health.

PRECONCEPTUAL PROGRAM

Nutritional considerations
✢ protein/amino acid deficiency
✢ essential fatty acid deficiency
✢ excess refined carbohydrates
✢ generalized vitamin and mineral deficiencies
✢ low body weight
✢ slimming diets
✢ previous P.M.S.
✢ previous use of contraceptive pill
✢ alcohol
✢ excess stimulants (tea and coffee)
✢ food additives
✢ food allergy/intolerance
✢ heavy metal (lead, mercury, cadmium, etc.) and pesticide toxicity – may need a detoxification diet but this should be undertaken well before getting pregnant

Maximize
✢ Intake of immune-boosting fruit and vegetables, antioxidant fruit and vegetables, ground mixed seeds.
Eat
✢ Some raw vegetables and sprouted seeds daily. Add carbohydrates such as quinoa, wheatgerm, and oatgerm, to salads and soups. Balance animal protein (fish and lean meat) with vegetable proteins.
Avoid
✢ Alcohol, stimulants, refined carbohydrates, hydrogenated and saturated fats, trans-fatty acids, additives, pesticides, allergens.

SUPPLEMENTS

A high-quality multivitamin/multimineral formula with good levels of all vitamins (except retinol; beta-carotene can be substituted), folic acid in particular, and also with minerals, especially zinc, magnesium, and iron; soy lecithin.

CAUTION

Any woman planning a pregnancy, whether or not she has a previous child with a birth defect, should always discuss diet and supplementation with her family physician before embarking on a self-help program.

GOOD LEVELS OF MINERALS AND VITAMINS HELP TO PRODUCE A HEALTHY BABY

GOOD BODY WEIGHT IN THE MOTHER INCREASES THE CHANCE OF A HEALTHY BABY

RIGHT *Nutritional changes, including adding fresh fruit and vegetables to the diet, may improve health during pregnancy and maximize the chance of producing a healthy baby.*

Pregnancy

OPTIMUM NUTRITION *can greatly improve your chances of having a healthy pregnancy, and a healthy baby. Since pregnancy is such a nutritionally demanding time for a woman, even the slightest deficiencies can have serious effects on the health of the baby. A healthy pregnancy will depend on a greater supply than normal of enough essential nutrients, vitamins, and minerals to meet the needs of the mother and the growing fetus.*

Today, more than ever before, miscarriage is the greatest threat to any pregnancy, with perhaps one in ten pregnant women miscarrying, and maybe as many as one in two where previous miscarriage has occurred. Also, since early miscarriages often go unnoticed or unreported, this is likely to be a gross underestimate. Many experts believe that miscarriage is a fairly good indication that a woman (or the father of her child) has been exposed to "environmental hazards". The list of such "hazards" is endless, but includes such things as smoking, alcohol intake, heavy metal toxicity, environmental pollutants (including pesticides, exhaust gases, etc.), plastics, stress, and suboptimum nutrition. All of these hazards need to be avoided as far as possible, in addition to maximizing intake of antioxidant nutrients (by food and/or as part of a multi-supplement), especially selenium, which is at high levels in Brazil nuts.

Environmental hazards have their most far-reaching effects in the very early stages of pregnancy, when cell division is most prolific – a time when many women do not even know they are pregnant.

Even seemingly innocuous substances can have a devastating effect. Very high levels of glucose in the diet are a common cause of blood-sugar swings, but during pregnancy high glucose levels have a more profound effect, interfering drastically with normal metabolism; they have been indicated in birth defects. The same problems do not occur with fructose (fruit sugar) and lactose (milk sugar).

During the first three months of pregnancy all the organs of the baby are completely formed. This is the period when optimum nutrition is most important. For some nutrients, the mother's blood supply offers the fetus only what can be spared. The mother may remain reasonably healthy, yet have very low levels of nutrients left over for the developing baby. It is even more important that good reserves have been built up by the mother preconceptually by following an optimum nutrition program, since these stores may dwindle quickly due to the common problem of "morning sickness".

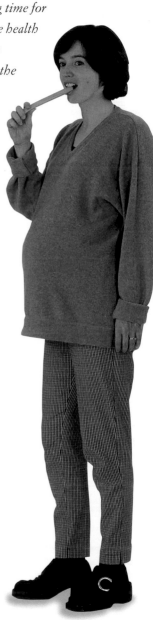

RIGHT *A good and regular intake of nutrients is vital throughout pregnancy.*

MINOR PROBLEMS IN PREGNANCY

Many minor problems can be prevented, or alleviated, by nutrition.

MILD ANEMIA

Iron-deficiency anemia may be present in 20 percent of pregnant women in a mild form, and your general physician may prescribe iron supplements. But it is as well to bear in mind that taking extra iron will depress zinc levels and may cause constipation. Zinc deficiency during the last two-thirds of pregnancy can alter the basic development of the fetal immune system and may cause hyperactivity and learning difficulties. Other nutrient deficiencies, including vitamin B_{12}, folic acid, manganese, and vitamin B_6 can also cause anemia. Insure that your diet contains extra wheatgerm, seeds (sesame, sunflower, pumpkin), and dark green vegetables.

CONSTIPATION

This may be due to iron supplements, but may also be the result of the fecal matter in the large intestine being more compressed because of the pressure from the developing baby. Drink plenty of fluids and eat fibrous fruit and vegetables, lentils, and beans. Avoid wheat bran.

LEG CRAMPS

Cramps are caused by muscles (usually in the calf) contracting strongly – going into "spasm". Deficiencies of calcium and/or magnesium may cause this to happen, so insure that you eat green leafy vegetables, nuts, and seeds (especially sesame).

STRETCH MARKS

If the skin loses its natural elasticity, stretch marks may develop and may be a sign of zinc deficiency. Good dietary sources of zinc are pumpkin seeds, fish, and shellfish. Additional vitamin C is needed to manufacture collagen, and is found in fresh fruit and vegetables. Vitamin E is involved in keeping skin supple; it is found in seed oils, cereals, seeds, and wheat-or oatgerm.

VARICOSE VEINS

These are caused by a restriction in the flow of blood from the feet and legs to a large vein in the groin area. Keep the venous system in good repair by eating a diet high in natural unprocessed foods, and supplying vitamin B-complex, vitamins C and E, and essential fatty acids.

KEEPING THE VEINS ELASTIC

Unlike most of the side effects of pregnancy, varicose veins will remain after the birth. However, veins can be kept free of the stiffening that makes them varicose with E.P.A. from oily fish, vitamin B₃ from poultry, and vitamin C from fruit and vegetables. The vegetables, together with nuts and seeds, also help avoid cramps.

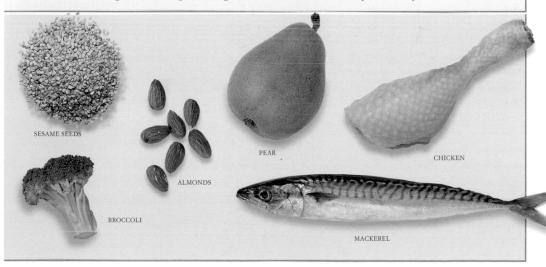

SESAME SEEDS

ALMONDS

PEAR

CHICKEN

BROCCOLI

MACKEREL

NUTRITIONAL CONSIDERATIONS DURING PREGNANCY

Upon conception, cells lining the uterus are stimulated to grow and divide rapidly. Similarly, rapid cellular division occurs in the developing embryonic tissue. In between cell divisions, the cell accumulates nutrients, especially amino acids and zinc. Both of these nutrients are, therefore, in great demand. Some estimates indicate that the requirements for vitamin B-complex, vitamin C, calcium, zinc, and magnesium increase by 30 to 100 percent during pregnancy. The intake of food as a whole, increases by around 15 to 20 percent.

In addition to the New Pyramid diet, the following are important.

❖ Have a ricecake, or take a small glass of apple juice, or ginger tea before rising to prevent nausea.

❖ Always eat breakfast – preferably a protein food such as yogurt.

❖ Eat five or six small meals a day and have some complex carbohydrate – choose from brown rice, buckwheat, barley, oats, fruit, pulses (legumes), or vegetables – along with a little protein – choose from fish, lean meat, or poultry, egg, yogurt, tofu, nuts, cottage or soy cheese – at each meal.

❖ If you have been advised to minimize your intake of mucus-forming foods, such as meat, eggs, and dairy produce, insure you obtain calcium from canned fish, tofu, vegetables, seeds, nuts, and pulses (legumes).

❖ Maximize your intake of fresh fruit and vegetables, and freshly ground seeds – sesame, sunflower, linseed (flax seed), and pumpkin.

NUTRITIONAL REQUIREMENTS DURING PREGNANCY

All nutrients are needed for a healthy pregnancy, just as they are at any time; the following are particularly important for the health of mother and baby.

NUTRIENT	REQUIRED FOR
Vitamin A	Fetal growth; visual development
Vitamin B6	Increased metabolism of protein
Vitamin B12	Red blood cell production; nervous system and brain
Folic acid	Manufacture of D.N.A. and red blood cells; proper neural tube development
Biotin	Manufacture of fatty acids; insuring B12 and folic acid are used properly
Vitamin C	Collagen production; oxygen carriage; immune boosting
Vitamin E	Oxygen carriage; protection of R.N.A. and D.N.A.; wound healing
Iron	Red blood cells/oxygen carriage
Calcium	Fetal skeleton
Magnesium	Fetal skeleton; metabolism; muscle activity
Zinc	Enzyme reactions; growth; functioning of D.N.A. and R.N.A.; antagonist to heavy metals
E.P.A./D.H.A. in fish oils; G.L.A. in evening primrose oil	Prostaglandins and cell membranes; brain development; retina of the eye

❖ Add wheat- or oatgerm to salads and soups.

❖ Eat some raw vegetables and sprouted seeds or pulses (legumes) each day.

❖ Minimize your intake of refined carbohydrate, sweet fruit and dried fruit, as well as tea, coffee, colas, and salt. Drink plenty of bottled water.

❖ Avoid alcohol, sugar, processed foods, additives, environmental pollutants, saturated and hydrogenated fat, soft cheeses, common food allergens, and trans-fatty acids.

NUTRITIONAL HELP FOR SERIOUS PROBLEMS IN PREGNANCY

There are several major ailments that need careful management.

PRE-ECLAMPSIA (TOXEMIA)

The first sign that pre-eclampsia (a condition in which the mother may have convulsions) may be occurring is a rise in blood pressure. This is usually accompanied by swelling of the ankles, caused by fluid retention, and protein appearing in the urine. These symptoms commonly begin during the last few weeks of pregnancy. The condition, which can normally be treated with bed rest and an optimum diet, can be very serious, so prenatal checkups are vital.

Incomplete formation of the placenta is one criterion related to pre-eclampsia, which is thought to interfere with an appropriate immune function in the mother. Some research has also implicated high copper levels, and this may be related to the usual drop in zinc in pregnancy. Additionally, there appears to be some evidence that low levels of vitamin B6 could predispose women to pre-eclampsia. It is advisable to insure good levels of calcium during pregnancy to protect against high blood pressure and toxemia.

Magnesium, because of its close biochemical relationship with calcium, has also been shown to prevent pre-eclampsia. Gamma linolenic acid (G.L.A.), given as evening primrose oil, has been useful for helping to treat high blood pressure

> ### CAUTION
> Publicity over the dangers of Listeria poisoning has focused on unpasturised milk products, but the bacterium can be found in pasteurized soft cheeses and pâtés too. Raw vegetables, fruit, and salads can also be contaminated.

in pre-eclampsia. High levels of zinc in the diet can help prevent many of the hypertensive problems – edema (water retention) and high blood pressure. Recent research has indicated that antioxidant supplementation during pregnancy clearly reduces the risk of pre-eclampsia.

Lastly, amino acids are crucial to proper fluid distribution in the body. Therefore, low protein intake may lead to hypertensive disorders, which may progress to pre-eclampsia – good protein intake is vital.

AFLATOXIN POISONING

This deadly substance is produced by molds that live on improperly stored pulses (legumes) and grains. Peanuts and beans that have been stored in damp climates are particularly at risk. Aflatoxins may cause mental retardation in the child, so ensure that these food items are obtained from a reputable source.

LISTERIA POISONING

Listeria monocytogenes is a bacterium that can grow well in chilled food, especially "prepared" meals. It is also common in unpasteurized

milk products, soft cheese, and pâtés. Babies who are infected by *Listeria,* which crosses the placental barrier, can be stillborn, or may develop septicemia with meningitis and/or pneumonia, within 48 hours of delivery.

Insure that refrigerators are working at the correct temperatures (below 39°F [4°C]). Avoid soft cheeses and pâtés, and carefully wash all vegetables and fruit that are to be eaten raw.

PROTEIN DEFICIENCY

Fetal development is the only period in a human being's life when new brain cells are being developed. A low-protein diet during this phase can stunt the development of the brain, as well as organ growth. A pregnant woman needs around an extra 1oz (25g) of protein daily. Insuring your diet contains sufficient protein is vital in the later stages of pregnancy when fetal growth is rapid.

PREMATURE LABOR

There is some evidence to suggest that taking calcium, manganese, and evening primrose oil regularly can be helpful in avoiding prematurity.

BELOW *Soft and unpasteurized cheeses are particularly prone to* Listeria *contamination.*

Breast Feeding

SOME RECENT RESEARCH *has indicated that children who are breastfed up to
a minimum of four months may have a reduced risk of high blood pressure, weight gain,
and circulatory problems in adulthood. If a mother can breast feed her baby, then she should
be given every encouragement to do so.*

Human milk is only going to be as good as the nutritional status of the mother, and if her diet has been anything less than optimum throughout her pregnancy, and even before, then there is a likelihood of her milk having suboptimum levels of nutrients. Moreover, we are all exposed to environmental toxins, even those of us who eat organic food, and some of these toxins are passed into breast milk and may cause problems in susceptible babies.

Yet certain trace elements, amino acids, and essential fatty acids are present in human breast milk that are not available in the same form elsewhere. For example, breast milk contains, among many other nutrients, selenium and chromium. Neither of these minerals is usually present in formula milks. The mineral manganese in breast milk is in a much more absorbable form than in formula milk, vitamin E is higher in breast milk, and the vitamin D is more active in preventing rickets. Present, also, are some of the mother's antibodies, which protect against certain infectious diseases during the first year of life. Breast milk tends to be deficient in zinc but, despite its lower levels, it is in a form that is much better absorbed than normal dietary zinc.

If you are unable to breast feed, choose the best formula milk you can find. Insure it does not contain added sugar or glucose. Compare the list of nutrient contents with other formula milks and choose the one that has the highest amounts of nutrients, especially the minerals zinc, chromium, selenium, and manganese.

BREAST MILK PASSES ON ANTI-
BODIES TO THE BABY THAT
STRENGTHENS ITS IMMUNE
SYSTEM AGAINST CONTRACTING
ALLERGIES

GIVING BABIES NON-HUMAN
MILKS CAN CAUSE ALLERGIES
OR DIETARY IMBALANCES

EVEN IF THE MOTHER
DOES NOT SUFFER FROM
FOOD INTOLERANCES
THEY CAN STILL OCCUR
IN THE BABY

LEFT *Food intolerances can
be passed on through breast
milk, although antibodies in
the milk can protect against
this occurring.*

PROBLEMS WITH BREAST FEEDING

The nutritional requirements of the mother are higher during breast feeding than at any other time. The nutrients that are required at higher levels are calcium, magnesium, iron, zinc, B vitamins, and folic acid. Breast milk contains a vitamin K-inhibiting substance and to insure that the baby is obtaining sufficient vitamin K in his or her breast milk, the mother needs to eat sufficient cauliflower and cabbage, which are high in vitamin K.

There is the possible problem of food allergy or intolerance developing as a result of the new infant reacting to allergens in the mother's milk. If defective genes are the root cause of allergy and intolerance, then we might expect most allergies to begin early in life, as indeed they do. A baby's immune system is not fully developed at birth, and to protect it against infection in the first few months of life, the mother's milk contains antibodies to common micro-organisms, bacteria, and viruses. The baby's gut is "leaky" to allow these antibodies through into its bloodstream. Due to this necessary degree of permeability, far more undigested food molecules also get into the blood than in an older child or adult. At the same time, the control reactions that regulate damaging immune reactions are not yet fully functioning. Any food that the baby eats or drinks during the first three months of life will be absorbed into the bloodstream in appreciable quantities. Some mechanisms, as yet poorly understood, prevent a baby from mounting a

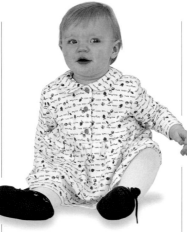

ABOVE *Some health problems in babies are a reaction to substances in their food.*

damaging reaction against its mother's breast milk proteins, although this can happen in extremely rare cases. Presumably this tolerance happens before birth while the baby is still in the womb. Because food molecules pass into breast milk from the mother's dietary intake, it is important for the mother to watch what she eats while breast feeding. It would be beneficial if she could eat a basic but varied hypoallergenic diet.

If a breastfed baby has eczema, skin problems, ear infections and blockage of the Eustachian tube, digestive problems, or problems sleeping, they are likely to be reacting to certain foods in the mother's diet. Cow's milk is a potential "allergen"

RIGHT *Breast milk is prone to being low in vitamin K, mothers should eat cauliflower and cabbage to improve the content.*

and can cause colic in breastfed babies. Others might be eggs, wheat, peanuts, some fish, some nuts, citrus, red wine, caffeine (in coffee, tea, colas, chocolate, etc.). The mother would be well advised to keep all major common food allergens out of her diet, and to note any consequent change in her infant's condition.

It is important that the mother's nutritional intake is not compromised in the process, and where a certain food, or group of foods, is removed from the diet, a good substitute should always be found. For example, if wheat is taken out, then rye, or other cereals can be used; soy or rice milk can be substituted in the mother's diet for cow's milk, or the mother may discover that although cow's milk produces digestive or skin reactions in her child, sheep's milk does not.

Nutritional therapists think that bottle-fed babies can escape the likelihood of intolerances if a rotation system is used for their formula milks. A typical rotation would be four days of cow's milk formula, followed by four days of soy milk formula, and then four days of goat's milk formula.

133

Optimum Nutrition for Babies and Children

BECAUSE BABIES AND *children are growing at a rapid rate, they are very susceptible to the effects of poor nutrition. Their immature immune systems and detoxification mechanisms make them more susceptible to infections, and pollution, toxins and additives in food. An optimum intake of nutrients will allow a child to have a well-nourished immune system, enabling them to throw off the common childhood infections much more quickly.*

While it may be beneficial for children to be exposed to a certain level of infections in order to prime the immune system, it is a different matter when considering pollutants and food allergens. Exposing very young children to such substances is not going to strengthen anything. You must insure that a breastfed infant is receiving, as far as it is possible, optimum, low-allergy, pollution-free nutrients in breast milk. This is done by paying attention to the mother's diet (see page 133). For children at the weaning stage, you should insure that common allergenic foods, such as wheat and citrus fruit, are not given as "first foods".

WEANING

Babies' teeth usually start to erupt at around six months, so this is probably a good time to start weaning. The baby may indicate that it is "weaning time" by demanding more milk feeds during the day or night. No baby should be given any "solid" food before the age of four months; there is a

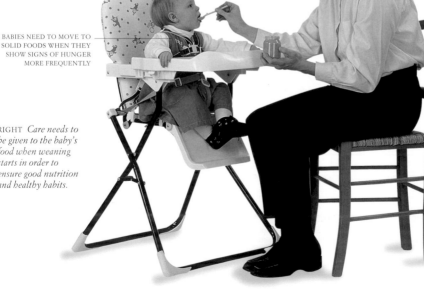

BABIES NEED TO MOVE TO SOLID FOODS WHEN THEY SHOW SIGNS OF HUNGER MORE FREQUENTLY

RIGHT *Care needs to be given to the baby's food when weaning starts in order to ensure good nutrition and healthy habits.*

likelihood of inducing food allergy before this time, due to immaturity of the digestive system.

Chewing on some solid food is a good way to encourage the teeth to come through properly. Avoid the wheat-based foods recommended for teething, and give the baby a crust of rye bread instead. If the parents eat a wholefood diet and the baby is encouraged to eat natural foods from the start, he/she will be more likely to fit in with the parents' meals as he gets older.

Prepared baby foods have improved enormously over the last ten years or so. It is now very likely that you will be able to choose from a range of baby foods that do not contain any artificial additives, sugar, cow's milk, or wheat, and are made from good wholesome organic ingredients. The important thing is to read the label carefully on all baby foods. If it contains cereal, it needs to be unrefined, and would be better if it were rice or oat cereal rather than wheat; plain white rice has a very low allergenicity and is highly digestible. Baby food should not contain added glucose, dextrose, sucrose, maltose, fructose, or modified starch, hydrolized protein, or any other chemical ingredient.

Despite the fact that one of the aims of infant feeding is to help babies to get to like the food you do, young children do not need the same amount of "fiber" as an adult. Soluble fibers found in apples, a little oatmeal, or rice pudding will be more than sufficient to keep their bowels working properly. At the start of weaning, children need foods that are very easily digested

As you proceed with weaning, continue to breast feed or give formula milk and introduce one new food into the child's diet every three or four days. Take note of any foods to which the child has any bad reaction – if high-protein allergenic food, like milk, wheat, or eggs are introduced into the diet too early (before ten months) they can set the stage for lifelong allergy.

WEANING FOODS
(In order of introduction to diet)

"Ancestral foods" (fruit, vegetables, seeds, nuts, fish) can be introduced first, and as each group is taken without problems, move onto the next. Leave wheat, potatoes, milk (especially cow's), and citrus fruit until later.

PURÉES	FRESH FOODS
✳ carrots	✳ banana, avocado, soft pear
✳ cauliflower	✳ peeled apple, raw carrot, cucumber
✳ mixed vegetable (e.g. carrot/cauliflower/turnip)	✳ creamed nuts (except peanuts), and creamed seeds (except sesame)
✳ different vegetable mixes (e.g. carrot/cauliflower/celery/beans)	✳ cooked lentils and haricot beans
✳ apple	✳ fish (well cooked – insure no bones/canned)
✳ mixed fruit purées (e.g. apple and banana)	✳ cooked white rice/rice flakes
✳ different vegetable mixes, now including potato	✳ cooked ground lamb, chicken or turkey
✳ soy milk yogurt	✳ cooked oats, barley flakes, rye bread – introduced one at a time
✳ cottage cheese	✳ other vegetables not yet used
✳ goat's milk custards	✳ oranges
✳ sheep's milk products	✳ wheat flakes, wholewheat bread, wheat cereal
	✳ cow's milk, and milk products
	✳ eggs
	✳ other "high allergenic" foods

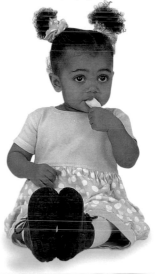

BELOW *Introduce new foods to your child gradually so that if any adverse reaction is experienced, it is easy to pinpoint the cause.*

Supplements for Children

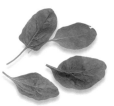

ABOVE *Spinach, eaten raw, is an excellent source of vitamins and minerals.*

T HERE IS INCREASING *evidence that poor diet not only affects children physically but also intellectually. A diet low in vitamins and minerals has been shown to affect behavior, as well as causing learning difficulties. Recent research has indicated that a high proportion of the children who are not receiving enough of the right nutrients for optimum brain function, are consuming a typical "Western diet". If you are concerned that your children are not receiving adequate vitamins and minerals, one solution is to give them a daily supplement.*

BABIES

Both breastfed babies and those on formula milks may have their "diets" supplemented with vitamin drops, which are available from the baby clinic, the pharmacy, or health food stores. These drops usually contain reasonable levels of vitamins A, C, and D, and will satisfy basic vitamin needs. Also available are various "drops" and "tonics" suitable for babies from six months to three years of age, which contain vitamins A and D, and several minerals (usually various salts) including iron, potassium, calcium, manganese, and copper. Yet to insure a child gets all the necessary nutrients (including minerals, vitamins, and essential fatty acids), a weaning program, started around six months of age, necessarily needs to include the foods as outlined for weaning.

YOUNG CHILDREN

When children have been used to fresh wholesome nourishment from birth, their diet will usually continue along the same lines, with occasional "hiccups" under peer pressure to eat junk food. If, however, you are a

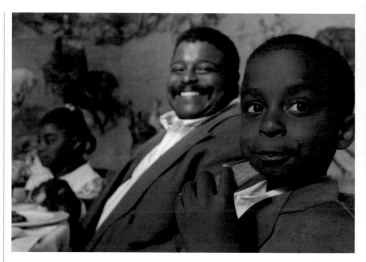

ABOVE *Insuring children establish a good cardiovascular system through diet is more important today, as our modern lifestyle means they exercise less.*

parent who came to nutritional healing a little after your babies became children, do not despair, simply encourage them, along with the rest of the family, to undertake the basics of the New Pyramid diet. Of particular importance is the type and level of fat eaten by growing children. No child should be eating great quantities of saturated or hydrogenated fat, or eating large amounts of sweet foods. Diets high in fat and sugar are just as bad for

children as they are for adults. This has recently been confirmed by results from an assessment of young children for cardiovascular fitness, which showed a great deterioration when compared to a survey taken two decades ago. However, young children do need a good supply of essential fatty acids for brain development, immune function, and general health, and these can be supplied by fish and wholefoods (especially seeds).

For growing children, the nutrients especially important include: vitamin A (for membrane integrity – protecting against infection); vitamin B-complex (for energy production, growth, brain and nerve development); vitamin C (good development of skin, connective tissue, and brain); calcium and magnesium (for healthy bones and teeth); zinc (for R.N.A. and D.N.A., and growth); fatty acids (proper cellular development, especially brain cells); and iron, chromium, selenium, and manganese.

SUPPLEMENTS FOR GROWING CHILDREN

Supplements available for young children contain a variety of vitamins and minerals, and usually include vitamins B6, folic acid, B12, pantothenic acid, iron, zinc, and iodine, in addition to those nutrients found in "baby" drops. Supplements are not given instead of a wholesome diet, but in addition to it, as "insurance" against disease and ill-health.

If you do decide to give your growing child a nutritional supplement, be very careful that you obtain a supplement correct for the age of your child, and do not be tempted to increase the dose if they decide on some days not to eat much. Children are more susceptible to vitamin toxicity than adults. Once a child reaches the age of around 12 years, they can usually take multicomplexes at adult doses, but consult with a nutritionist or your physician first.

FOOD ALLERGIES AND HYPERACTIVITY

Food allergies can result in a vast range of different symptoms. The most common in children are asthma, eczema, behavioral problems, and hyperactivity (attention deficit disorder). Asthma and eczema are commonly caused by cow's milk products, eggs, wheat, or citrus. But symptoms that have a degree of emotional/intellectual involvement can be caused by food allergens that are less easy to spot.

Behavioral problems manifest themselves in temper tantrums, self-inflicted damage, poor verbal communication, fearlessness, impulsiveness, short attention span, and egocentricity. Behavioral problems can totally destroy family life. Conventional medicine uses a variety of sedative drugs, which may temporarily calm the symptoms, but do not heal the cause.

More boys seem to suffer than girls, and many seem to have a high level of copper in their bodies, which automatically raises the need for zinc – vital for proper brain function. It is possible to use the criteria of nutritional healing to get to the root of these common problems.

RASPBERRIES

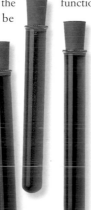

TOP *Hyperactivity benefits from a diet that omits fruits containing salicylates.*

LEFT *Food colorings – many of which are linked with hyperactivity – should be avoided.*

HYPERACTIVITY AND BEHAVIORAL PROBLEMS

Nutritional considerations
✛ low intake of protein
✛ fruits high in salicylates and sugar
✛ refined carbohydrates
✛ low intake of zinc
✛ food additives, flavorings, colors, preservatives, monosodium glutamate, aspartame
✛ environmental pollutants
　✛ food allergy/intolerance
　✛ caffeine (colas, chocolate – also tea and coffee if consumed)
　✛ heavy metal toxicity
　✛ generalized mineral and vitamin deficiencies (especially B3, B6, biotin, zinc, and magnesium
✛ hypoglycemia
✛ low levels of essential fatty acids
Maximize
✛ Intake of vegetables and non-salicylate fruit (e.g. bananas, mango), and mixed seeds (sesame, pumpkin, sunflower, linseed).
Balance
✛ Animal protein with vegetable protein and carbohydrates.
Eat
✛ Plenty of fiber from brown rice, and small amounts of oats and/or rye, fruit and vegetables (cellulose and pectins).

SUPPLEMENTS

A high-quality children's formula with good levels of vitamin B-complex (especially B1, B3, B6, and B12), vitamin C, vitamin E, calcium, magnesium, zinc, chromium, iron, iodine, and selenium; essential fatty acids – evening primrose oil (or starflower oil) and whole fish body oil; Ginkgo biloba.

137

Adolescence and Menopause

ADOLESCENCE IS A *time when children are likely to spend their hard-earned pocket money on chips and candy. Providing a nourishing evening meal (containing a good balance of high-quality protein and vegetables), for all the family to eat together, insures that at least some daily nutrient standards are being met. A suboptimum diet in menopause can lead to adrenal gland exhaustion, hypoglycemia, and stress, bringing on distressing menopausal symptoms.*

NUTRITIONAL CONSIDERATIONS DURING ADOLESCENCE

Recent work in the U.S.A. on child vandals and older offenders claims that a poor diet high in sugar (in particular), refined and processed foods, and low in fresh wholefoods, has a direct effect on the times an offender commits a crime. Some researchers also claim that juvenile delinquents, unresponsive to counseling, became more "counselable" when provided with essential fatty acid-rich oils.

The additional problems of adolescence are usually focused around increased hormone production, which may temporarily disrupt metabolism. This is also the age of "growth spurts". Adolescents need a high level of good-quality protein, complex carbohydrates (and if they refuse many of the vegetables you offer them, at least give them wholegrains, pasta, rice, and bread), and adequate vitamins and minerals for their growth. One mineral commonly deficient in these years is zinc, especially if the young adult is not keen on vegetables, shellfish, or seeds. Low intakes of zinc, and other minerals, are said by some therapists to be associated both with "teenage spots" and acne.

Much more problematic are the eating disorders that afflict adolescent girls, convinced that they are fat, no matter how slim they really are. Both anorexia and bulimia nervosa are primarily psychological disorders focusing on issues of control and self-punishment.

Zinc deficiencies can play a key role in bizarre eating behavior, in particular the level of appetite – one of the functions of zinc is to help maintain a healthy appetite. Zinc has been shown to improve the appetite and attitudes of anorexics, as well as children who are "picky" eaters and the elderly.

Insuring children of prepubescent age eat well, and consume foods high in zinc in particular, is an excellent grounding for good eating. Girls, in particular, should be encouraged to eat zinc-rich foods such as pumpkin seeds.

RIGHT *Good nutrition is especially important in adolescence, but hard to achieve.*

NUTRITIONAL CONSIDERATIONS DURING MENOPAUSE

The emergence of menopausal symptoms is related to change in hormonal status as a woman reaches the end of her childbearing years. In a healthy woman, a backup system of estrogen circulation helps to maintain a portion of the secondary sexual characteristics required to remain feminine. When this backup system starts to fail – possibly the result of poor nutrition – menopausal symptoms such as hot flashes, sweating, headaches, loss of libido, vaginal dryness etc. occur.

Hot flashes may be the result of an allergic reaction, caused by an increased toxic load on the body, for which many nutritionists recommend a hypoallergenic diet. The more severe the intolerant reactions to foods, the greater the likelihood of essential nutrient deficiencies being present.

HORMONE REPLACEMENT THERAPY

Hormone replacement therapy is hormonal replacement to delay menopause. It involves the administration of estrogen and sometimes synthetic progesterone.

Many studies do indicate a real benefit from H.R.T. in terms of decreased menopausal symptoms. It is well known that estrogen decreases hot flashes and vaginal dryness, but unfortunately it can also cause weight gain, bloating, and irritability.

Mostly, H.R.T. merely postpones symptoms of the menopause. It alters the bal-

ance of vitamins and minerals and has been linked to cardiovascular disease, strokes, and cancers of the uterus and breast. Taking hormones also puts the liver under stress as it strives to detoxify them.

Current research indicates that natural hormones can counter menopausal symptoms, and reduce the risk of osteoporosis and heart

disease. The adaptogenic herbs, such as Agnus castus and Dong quai, have been used for centuries to balance hormonal levels, prevent hot flashes, and relieve psychological smptoms. Vitamin E has many benefits; it helps prevent hot flashes, reduces the risk of heart disease, and protects the skin against aging. Evening primrose oil and fish oils can help protect against heart disease and strokes.

MENOPAUSAL SYMPTOMS

Nutritional considerations
✛ low intake of zinc and other important micronutrients (calcium, magnesium, vitamin B-complex, vitamin D, vitamin E, and E.F.A.s)
✛ toxicity
✛ food allergy/intolerance
✛ refined carbohydrates and sugar (causing hypoglycemia)
✛ excess stimulants (tea, coffee, alcohol)
✛ poor intake of nutrients generally or poor absorption
✛ low stomach acid

Maximize
✛ Intake of fresh vegetables and fruit (organic whenever possible), vegetable protein, especially tofu and other soy products, pulses (legumes), nuts, seeds, and seed vegetables (green beans, etc.). Eat plenty of ground mixed seeds (sesame, sunflower, pumpkin, and linseed).

Eat
✛ Wheatgerm or oatgerm on your salads and soups. Use cold-pressed olive oil on salads for extra vitamin E.
✛ Eat at least some raw vegetables and sprouted seeds daily.
✛ Use fructose to sweeten drinks and foods. Drink plenty of bottled or filtered water between meals.

Avoid
✛ Refined carbohydrates, sugar, processed food, saturated and hydrogenated fats, trans-fatty acids, food additives and pollutants, and allergens.

SUGGESTED SUPPLEMENTS

A high-potency multivitamin/multimineral complex containing good levels of vitamins A, B-complex (especially B5 and B6), C, and E, calcium, magnesium, zinc, iodine, and selenium; bioflavonoids (such as hesperidin); essential fatty acids (evening primrose oil and fish oils); royal jelly; kelp; Siberian ginseng; Aloe vera juice; lecithin; wild yam extract; Agnus castus; blackcurrant seed oil; Dong quai; gamma-oryzanol; digestive enzymes. A probiotic supplement, such as Lactobacillus acidophilus, may be required for yeast overgrowth.

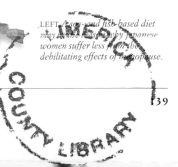

LEFT A soy- and fish-based diet may be the reason why Japanese women suffer less from the debilitating effects of menopause.

Useful Addresses

AUSTRALIA

Australian College of Nutritional & Environmental Medicine
13 Hilton Street
Beaumaris
Victoria 3193
Tel: 9589 6088.

CANADA

National Institute of Nutrition
2565 Carling Avenue, Suite 400
Ottawa, Ontario
Canada K1Z 8RI
Tel: (613) 235 3355

NEW ZEALAND

New Zealand Natural Health Practitioners Accreditation Board
P.O. Box 37 – 491
Auckland

U.K.

B.A.N.T.
(British Association of Nutritional Therapists)
27 Old Gloucester Street
London
WC1W 3XX
Tel: (0870) 606 1284

The Breakspear Hospital
Lord Alexander House
Water House Street
Hemel Hempstead
Herts HP1 1DL
Tel: (01442) 261333

Bristol Cancer Help Center
Grove House
Cornwallis Grove
Clifton
Bristol BS8 4PG
Tel: (0117) 9809 505

British Society for Allergy and Environmental Medicine
P.O. Box 28
Totton
Southampton
Hants SO40 2ZA
Tel: (023) 8081 2124

Community Health Foundation
188 Old Street
London EC1V 9FR
Tel: 020 7251 4076

Eating Disorders Association
1st Floor
Wensum House
103 Prince of Wales Road
Norwich NR1 1DW
Tel: (01603) 621414

The Hyperactive Children's Support Group
71 Whyke Lane
Chichester
West Sussex
PO19 2LD

Institute for Optimum Nutrition (I.O.N.)
Blades Court
Deodar Road
London SW15 2NU
Tel: 020 8877 9993

U.S.

American Academy of Environmental Medicine
4510 W. 89th Street
Prairie Village
KS 66207
Tel: (913) 341 3625

American College of Advancement in Medicine
P.O. Box 3427
Laguna Hills
CA 92654
Tel: (714) 583 7666

American Dietetic Association
216 W. Jackson Blvd.
Suite 800
Chicago
IL 60606
Tel: (312) 899 0040

American Preventive Medical Association
275 Millway
P.O. Box 732
Barnstable
MA 02630
Tel: (508) 362 4343

Linus Pauling Institute
440 Page Mill Road
Palo Alto
CA 94306-2031
Tel: (415) 327 4064

Acknowledgments

With thanks to:

Mary Armstrong, Janine Bennett, Jacob Bevis, Patricia Blunt, Philip Constable, Paul Golding, Alexandra Grant, Debbie Grant, Sally Hardy, Sam Hollingdale, Louise Inch, Alastair Mackay, Derek Ockmore, Helen Omand, Donna Paplett, Georgette Rae, Sharon Rashand, Abiola Roberts, Ajebowale Roberts, Carolyn Jikiemi Roberts, Michele Sawyer, Andrew Stemp, Rebecca Vesti-Nielsen, Beth Webster, Louise Williams, and also Solutions and Courts for help with photography.

Picture credits:

GettyOneStone: pp: 18, 23, 33CBR, 40B, 41T; *Image Bank*: pp: 9T, 50T, 66, 70, 79, 136; *Nasa*: p.40T; *Science Photo Library*: pp: 13BR, 28TR, 48.

Further Reading

General Nutrition

JAMES F. BALCH M.D. AND PHYLLIS A. BALCH, *Prescription for Nutritional Healing* Avery Publishing Group Inc., 1990.

JEFFREY S. BLAND PH.D. WITH SARA H. BENUM M.A., *Genetic Nutritioneering* Keats Publishing, 1999.

UDO ERASMUS, *Fats that Heal, Fats that Kill,* Alive books, 1993.

Prescription for change: Health and the Environment, Friends of the Earth, 1995.

JOE AND TERESA GRAEDON, *The People's Guide to Deadly Drug Interactions,* St. Martin's Press, 1995.

DR ANTHONY LEEDS, JENNIE BRAND MILLER, KAYE FOSTER-POWELL, DR STEPHEN COLAGIURI, *The Glucose Revolution,* Hodder and Stoughton 1998.

LINDA LAZARIDES, *The Principles of Nutritional Therapy,* Thorsons, 1996.

MARIA LINDER, *Nutritional Biochemistry and Metabolism,* Appleton and Lange, 1991.

KATHY MATTHEWS AND ROBERT M. GILLER, *Natural Prescriptions: Dr Giller's Natural Treatments and Vitamin Therapies for More Than 100 Common Ailments,* Ballantine Books, 1995.

DENISE MORTIMORE, *The Complete Illustrated Guide to Vitamins and Minerals,* Thorsons, 2001.

DENISE MORTIMORE, *In a Nutshell. Nutritional Healing,* Element Books, 1999.

MICHAEL MURRAY AND JOSEPH PIZZORNO, *Encyclopaedia of Natural Medicine,* Macdonald & Co., 1992.

DR. MELVYN R. WERBACH, *Healing through Nutrition,* HarperCollins, 1995

MELVYN WERBACH M.D., *Nutritional Influences on Illness,* Third Line Press, 1996.

RAY C. WUNDERLICH M.D., *Natural Alternatives to Antibiotics,* Keats Publishing, 1995.

Specific Needs/Conditions

MARTIN L. BUDD, *Low Blood Sugar (Hypoglycemia),* Thorsons, 1987.

LEON CHAITOW N.D. D.O. AND NATASHA TRENEV, *Probiotics,* Thorsons, 1990.

DR. MICHAEL COLGAN, *Optimum Sports Nutrition,* Advanced Research Press, 1993.

SANDRA GOODMAN PH.D., *Nutrition and Cancer,* Green Library Publications, 1995.

LESLIE KENTON, *Lean Revolution: Eat more to shed fat the energy way,* Ebury Press, 1994.

DR. P. KINGSLEY AND IAN STOAKES, *The Nutron Diet,* Penguin, 1994.

ALAN E. LEWIS AND DALLAS CLOUATRE PH.D., *Melatonin and the Biological Clock,* Keats Publishing, 1996.

KATE NEIL, *Balancing Hormones Naturally,* I.O.N. Press, 1994.

ALEXANDER SCHAUSS PH.D. AND CAROLYN COSTIN M.A. M.F.C.C., *Anorexia and Bulimia,* Keats Publishing, 1997.

PATSY WESTCOTT, *Thyroid Problems,* Thorsons, 1995.

Diets/Cookbooks

JILL CARTER AND ALISON EDWARDS, *The Rotation Diet Cookbook,* Element Books, 1997.

JACK CHALLEM AND VICTORIA DOLBY, *The Health Benefits of Soy* Keats Publishing, 1996.

RITA GREER, *Wheat, Milk and Egg-Free Cooking* Thorsons, 1989.

PETTA JANE GULLIVER, *Food Children Enjoy,* Cornish Connection, 1992.

MICHAEL VAN STRATEN AND BARBARA GRIGGS, *Super Fast Foods,* Dorling Kindersley, 1994.

MICHAEL VAN STRATEN AND BARBARA GRIGGS, *The Super Foods Diet Book,* Dorling Kindersley, 1992.

XANDRIA WILLIAMS, *Overcoming Candida: The Ultimate Cookery Guide,* Element Books, 1998.

Index

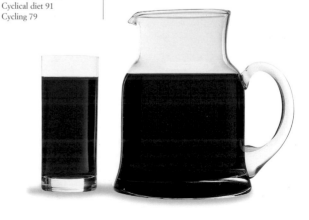

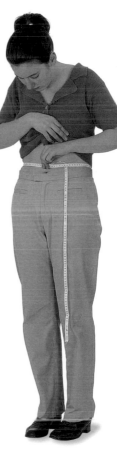

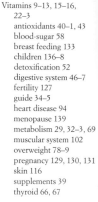